DASH DIET

For Beginners

Lower Blood Pressure, Reduce Cholesterol
and Manage Diabetes Naturally

Table of Contents

FREE BONUS MATERIAL

Thank you for reading this book. I hope you find it insightful and helpful. To help my readers I've put together additional health and fitness resources:

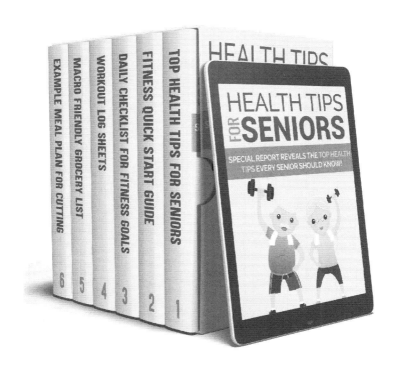

1. **Top Tips for Seniors** to enjoy your life and avoid health problems as you age

2. **6 Step Quick Start Guide** to finally take your fitness under control

3. **Daily Checklist** to stay on track with your fitness goals

4. **Workout Log Sheet** for keeping track of your workouts

5. **Macro Friendly Grocery List** to never run out of ideas what to eat

6. **Example Meal Plan** to supercharge your fat loss

To get your bonuses go to link:
http://bit.ly/4oMJRRK

or scan QR code
with your camera

Introduction

The fact that you are here shows that you have taken a bold step to do something about your health – the most important thing in your life. Congratulations.

In recent years, we've become all too dependent on the pharmaceutical industry for our health. We've come to believe that we can pop a pill to solve any health problem and have failed to take responsibility for our own decisions. Many common health problems, including serious diseases such as diabetes, heart disease, and cancer, have been thought to be a "normal," part of aging.

What if the real story was completely different and you had control over many of your long term health outcomes? Yes, aging and death will get us all in the end – but you can choose to be healthy and age well or you can sacrifice your health to diseases believed to be "inevitable" and become a prisoner to drugs and endless doctor visits.

You are what you eat; how well your body functions is highly dependent on what you put in your mouth. We now know that nutrition can influence whether or not you develop dementia or Alzheimer's disease, as well as how well you can get around and take care of yourself when you're elderly.

Some things are indeed genetic and your family history might loom large. Even then, taking control of your diet and nutrition will go a long way toward promoting your overall health. You are not a victim and the fact that you've chosen to read this book indicates you're ready to take charge of your own health!

So, why is the DASH Diet important and something you should consider trying? The answer is simple. DASH was originally developed specifically to deal with high blood pressure or hypertension, but it turns out that multiple health issues such as being overweight, developing diabetes and many of the other issues that we've already mentioned are all related. At their root, they at least in part, have a common cause. So while DASH had a specific intent – to lower blood pressure – it also improves health across the board, promoting weight loss, improving blood sugar, and reducing cholesterol. In addition, in recent years, evidence has linked high blood sugars to cancer (lots of insulin in your bloodstream contributes as well). Since DASH helps you lose weight, it may even lessen chances of cancer.

Enough of the pep talk. It's time to get started. Let's find out what the DASH Diet is all about, how and why it was developed, and how you can use it to improve your health!

Chapter 1. Know your risk for high blood pressure

Hypertension is an alternative name for high blood pressure. It can lead to severe health problems and increase the risk of heart disease, stroke, and sometimes even death. Keeping blood pressure under control is vital for preserving health and reducing the risk of these dangerous conditions. In this chapter, we examine factors that can cause high blood pressure.

Up to a billion people are estimated to have high blood pressure. It's more acute in developed countries and when we examine possible causes of high blood pressure, the reasons why become clear. In the United States, it is estimated that about half of all adults are suffering from high blood pressure, but many are not aware of this fact. The actual number is unknown and it's often called "the silent killer" as someone can appear to be completely healthy and yet have high blood pressure. Their body may look fine from the outside, but internally, it's being destroyed, minute by minute.

As mentioned earlier, in many cases, high blood pressure can be due to family history or genetics. However, many environmental factors can contribute as well. This, coupled with your lifestyle choices, may work for or against you. If we assume that high blood pressure exists in your family and then you adopt an unhealthy lifestyle of smoking or not maintaining a healthy weight through diet and exercise, then the chances are high that you are staring down the barrel of hypertension.

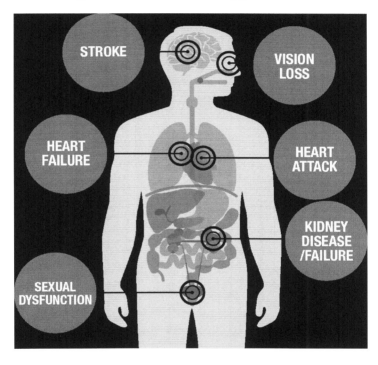

Health Threats From Hypertension
(source: www.heart.org)

Some of the most common causes that have been identified include:

Smoking

Cigarette smoking, in particular, has been strongly identified as an environmental risk factor for developing high blood pressure. This is due to the fact that people who smoke cigarettes get higher amounts of nicotine in their system.

Weight gain/obesity

Not all overweight people have high blood pressure, but it's clear that being overweight significantly increases your risk of developing it. The heavier you get, the higher the risk.

Sedentary lifestyle

Exercise counteracts hypertension. It helps keep the blood vessels flexible and responsive and helps keep the heart in shape. Someone who has good cardiovascular fitness has a lower resting heart rate and their heart pumps with a healthier level of force, so the blood pressure is reduced as compared to what it would be otherwise. In contrast, people who don't exercise raise their risk of developing high blood pressure, especially if they have a family history.

Race

Studies indicate that African Americans are more prone to high blood pressure than other groups. However, bear in mind that all racial and ethnic groups have plenty of risk of high blood pressure and its victims include people of all races and from every country across the globe.

Kidney disease

The kidneys are closely tied to the healthy maintenance of blood sugar. They help regulate the amount of fluid and salt in the body. When you are suffering from kidney disease, the kidneys may not function as well and this may lead to fluid and sodium retention, which can cause high blood pressure.

Age

Simply getting older raises risk, although we would never call high blood pressure "normal." However, as you get older, things don't work as well (you knew that, right?). If your joints are stiffening, you can bet your arteries are as well. Even though you may be reasonably healthy overall, simply getting older raises your risk of developing some level of high blood pressure. There is some debate about whether older people need to use the same standards as to what constitutes a diagnosis of hypertension or not, but a general rule applies. You're better off if your blood pressure is below 140/100.

Nutritional deficiencies

Nutritional deficiencies of potassium and magnesium can lead to the development of high blood pressure, along with other health problems such as heart palpitations and muscle cramps. Salt, especially in excess causes your body to retain fluid as the body adapts to maintain a healthy balance of sugar levels. Salt also promotes the contraction of blood vessels, among other things. All of these factors can lead to high blood pressure.

In Summary

The DASH Diet provides an opportunity to address several items on this list. It reduces salt in the diet and addresses nutritional deficiencies of potassium and magnesium. The practice of consuming large amounts of fruit and vegetables, along with a low-fat diet reduces the risk of kidney problems. Controlling weight can also reduce the risks of developing high blood pressure.

Chapter 2. Why you should go on the DASH Diet

What Is the DASH Diet?

DASH is an acronym used to refer to "Dietary Approaches to Stop Hypertension." The DASH eating plan is well researched and recommended by a number of reputable health organizations within the United States. The DASH Diet aims to address dietary patterns that can reduce symptoms of hypertension and even prevent such diseases.

The DASH Diet eating plan includes a variety of fruits and vegetables as well as low-fat dairy products and whole grains. Proteins include poultry, fish, red meat and nuts. Limited amounts of sweets are permitted within the plan. Following this healthy balanced eating approach benefits overall as well as specific health concerns such as hypertension.

The DASH Diet was developed by the National Institute of Health as they compared several eating plans and their impact on blood pressure or hypertension.

It was discovered that the DASH eating plan had a significant impact on systolic blood pressure as well as diastolic blood pressure. Researchers found that this particular eating plan was very effective in reducing symptoms of hypertension.

Hypertension is a widespread condition impacting millions of people worldwide. This straightforward, easy to implement eating plan provides a road to improved overall health, including a lessening of hypertension symptoms.

Sodium and Hypertension

Our kidneys function is to remove extra fluids from the body after filtering the blood. The extra fluid is directed to the bladder and eliminated from the body as urine. This process uses osmosis, which requires a delicate balance of potassium and sodium.

Eating excess sodium, which is basically the salt in your diet, disrupts this balance, compromising the effectiveness of your kidneys in eliminating the fluids.

Munching on salty food causes you to pee less frequently. In fact, before a long journey or when going to a function where the bathroom is not readily accessible, some people will eat a pinch of salt and this will effectively keep their bladder from filling for hours.

While such one-off instances may be harmless, a constant intake of sodium raises blood pressure due to the excess fluid. The strain put on the kidneys can lead to kidney disease, which will, in turn, cause toxins to accumulate in the body. The arteries are affected as well. The extra blood pressure caused by the excess fluid strains the arteries and the tiny muscles in their walls become thicker while attempting to keep up with the pumping. Thicker muscles mean that the space inside the arteries is reduced, raising the blood pressure even higher as it is now being forced through a constricted space.

For these reasons, there is a specific version of the DASH Diet that pays precise attention to the amount of salt in the diet, recommending a maximum of 2,300 mg of sodium a day. If you're already suffering from hypertension, your daily limit should not exceed 1,500 mg. Note that the average American's diet consists of up to 3,400 mg of sodium in a single day.

Even when you do not add a single grain of salt to your food, there's already so much of it in processed foods. This is one of the reasons why the DASH Diet highly recommends fresh foods.

You can reduce your sodium intake by getting a substitute for table salt in your food. There are several natural spices such as ginger or garlic that have that sour tinge that you crave for in salt. Another alternative is to sprinkle fresh lemon juice, especially on meat.

Rinse canned foods before cooking. Most of them come soaked with a salty sauce which you can do away with. How about processed meat? Check the labels for sodium content. Sausages, hot dogs, bacon, ham, and the like tend to be quite salty. If you cannot find a sodium-free/low option, stay away from them altogether. Finally, remove that salt shaker from the dinner table. Sometimes the act of adding salt is purely psychological, with some people adding even before they taste the food. Even in a restaurant, ask the waiter to take it back. Once it's out of sight, chances are, you won't even need it.

History of the DASH Diet

The DASH Diet dates back to the early 1990s when concern was raised about the prevalence of lifestyle diseases, among them hypertension. In 1992, under the funding of the National Institute of Health (NIH), several research projects were initiated to determine if dietary changes could be effective in treating hypertension.

The participants were provided with a meal plan and advised not to include any other lifestyle modification so that all the changes could be attributed directly to the dietary interventions.

The results were encouraging. A decrease of about 6 to 11 mm / Hg was reported in systolic blood pressure in a span of a few weeks. Lower levels of sodium in the diet correlated with lower blood pressure levels. In addition to reducing hypertension, cholesterol levels were reduced as well.

After several subsequent studies and experiments with positive results, the DASH Diet became and still is, highly recommended as a long-term remedy for hypertension.

Benefits of the DASH Diet

For a diet that was formulated to treat hypertension and which in most cases, has successfully done so, the DASH Diet has so many additional benefits. As it is basically healthy eating, the body benefits in multiple aspects. Even if you're not suffering from high blood pressure, the DASH Diet is still highly recommended. It'll go a long way in helping you avoid the condition as well as other lifestyle diseases such as diabetes, obesity, and heart disease.

If you're already suffering from hypertension, this diet can help you ease the symptoms which include headaches, chest pains, fatigue, labored breathing, and irregular heartbeat. Even if you're already on medication, the dietary changes recommended by this diet will regulate your blood pressure, so you don't have to live on medication.

Additional benefits include:

More Nutritious Meals

Eliminating processed foods and incorporating more fresh foods gives you healthy meals which are beneficial for every aspect of your wellbeing. Adjusting may take some effort at first, especially if you're accustomed to fast foods, but the results will be well worth the effort. You will reduce the chances of health issues throughout your lifetime and enjoy a largely vibrant, pain-free life.

Healthier Kidneys

The nutrients found in the DASH eating plan, including potassium, calcium, magnesium, and fiber, nourish every part of the body, and the kidneys are no exception. The lower consumption of sodium as recommended, further favor the kidneys, allowing them to filter blood efficiently.

Cardiovascular Health

The DASH Diet decreases your consumption of refined carbohydrates by increasing your consumption of foods high in potassium and dietary fiber (fruits, vegetables, and whole grains). It also lessens your consumption of saturated fats. Therefore, the DASH Diet has a positive effect on your lipid profile and glucose tolerance, which reduces the prevalence of metabolic syndrome (MS) in post-menopausal women.

Reports state that a diet limited to 500 calories favors a loss of 17% of total body weight in 6 months in overweight women. This reduces the prevalence of metabolic syndrome by 15%. However, when this diet follows the patterns of the DASH Diet, while triglycerides decrease similarly, the reduction in weight and blood pressure is even greater.

It also reduces blood sugar and increases HDL (high-density lipoprotein cholesterol), which decreases the prevalence of MS in 35% of women. These results contrasted with those of other studies, which have reported that the DASH Diet alone, i.e., without caloric restriction, does not affect HDL and glycemia. This means that the effects of the DASH Diet on MS are associated mainly with the greater reduction in BP (Blood Pressure) and that, for more changes, the diet would be required to be combined with weight loss.

Helpful for Patients with Diabetes

The DASH Diet helps reduce inflammatory and coagulation factors (C-reactive protein and fibrinogen) in patients with diabetes. These benefits are associated with the contribution of antioxidants and fibers, given the high consumption of fruits and vegetables that the DASH Diet requires. In addition, the DASH Diet has been shown to reduce total cholesterol and LDL (low-density lipoprotein cholesterol), which reduces the estimated 10-year cardiovascular risk. Epidemiological studies have determined that women in the highest quintile of food consumption, according to the DASH Diet, have a 24% to 33% lower risk of coronary events and an 18% lower risk of a cerebrovascular event. Similarly, a meta-analysis of six observational studies has determined that the DASH Diet can reduce the risk of cardiovascular events by 20%.

Weight Reduction

Limited research associates the DASH Diet, in isolation, with weight reduction. In some studies, weight reduction was greater when the subject was on the DASH Diet as compared to an isocaloric controlled diet. This could be related to the higher calcium intake and lower energy density of the DASH Diet. The American guidelines for the treatment of obesity emphasize that, regardless of diet, a caloric restriction would be the most important factor in reducing weight.

However, several studies have made an association between greater weight and fat loss in diets and caloric restriction and higher calcium intake. Studies have also observed an inverse association between dairy consumption and body mass index (BMI). In obese patients, weight loss has been reported as being 170% higher after 24 weeks on a hypocaloric diet with high calcium intake.

In addition, the loss of trunk fat was reported to be 34% of the total weight loss as compared to only 21% in a control diet. It has also been determined that a calcium intake of 20 mg per gram has a protective effect in overweight middle-aged women. This would be equivalent to 1275 mg of calcium for a western diet of 1700 kcal.

Despite these reports, the effect that diet-provided calcium has on women's weight after menopause is a controversial subject. An epidemiological study has noted that a sedentary lifestyle and, to a lesser extent, caloric intake is associated with post-menopausal weight gain and calcium intake is not associated with it. The average calcium intake in this group of women is approximately 1000 mg, which would be low, as previously stated. Another study of post-menopausal women shows that calcium and vitamin D supplementation in those with a calcium intake of less than 1200 mg per day decreases the risk of weight gain by 11%.

In short, the DASH Diet has positive impacts, both in weight control and in the regulation of fatty tissue deposits, due to its high calcium content (1200 mg/day). The contribution of calcium plays a vital role in the regulation of lipogenesis.

Drawbacks of the Dash Diet

Sodium Intake Control

The average American consumes 3,400 milligrams of sodium. This is according to the Center for Disease Control.

The DASH Diet program requires one to adjust and cut your salt intake to 2300 milligrams of sodium per day. Potentially, one should adjust to 1,500 milligrams per day.

That adjustment won't come easy to those who eat a typical American diet.

Most of the sodium consumed in a typical American diet comes from heavily processed foods. Even for those that are not reliant on processed food, the adjustment to lower sodium intake won't be easy.

Not letting go of the salt shaker is one of the main reasons why most people struggle.

A study investigating compliance with the diet has shown that people see it as a big challenge to stick to the program. They need more than counseling to stick to it.

According to researchers, the intake of dietary fat in the program goes a long way to help people stick to the diet.

Dash Diet is not the Cheapest

The fact that the diet relies on fresh fruits and vegetables can make it expensive. Fresh meat and seafood are never cheap too.

If you also consider that fresh fruits and vegetables go bad faster; there is a high likelihood of food waste when on the DASH Diet.

The option of canned or frozen foods is cheaper although preserved fruits and vegetables may contain added sugars and sodium.

The way to challenge this con is by careful planning. Taking the time to plan ahead, creating proper meal plans that incorporate seasonal produce and of course buying the foods in bulk, are all smart moves and practices to minimize the overall cost of the diet program.

They also help you stick to the diet in the long run. Your body will be around a lot longer than that expensive handbag. Invest in yourself. In the same way that cheap fuel will wreck your car, cheap processed food will wreck your body and will only cost you more in medical bills.

No Convenience Foods

The DASH Diet often doesn't include the luxury of take-out or delivery. There are no meals that can be ordered to be conveniently delivered to your doorstep as some of the other diets (e.g., Atkins Diet). The DASH Diet does not have the convenience of pre-measured portions and meals and snacks that are ready to eat. At the frozen section of the stores, there are no pre-cooked foods that fit the requirements of the diet.

Simply put, the DASH is not a commercial diet. With it, you have to get up and work for your meal.

No Organized Support

Any other popular characteristic of some food regimens is support groups; most of the other popular diet programs provide face-to-face counseling, institution meetings, or peer-to-peer coaching. These functions assist people in getting through rough patches when their motivation has waned. It also provides them with the opportunity to ask questions and learn insightful recommendations and insider hints.

At the same time, as you will discover, plenty of DASH Diet information is readily available. Unfortunately, there's rarely an organized support platform for the plan.

However, don't be discouraged. The way to deal with this is to approach any registered dietician as they are all too familiar with this eating plan.

Most dieticians would be willing to help you to broaden your meal plans or offer training and guide while you need it.

Requires Food Tracking

There is no calorie counting required on this diet per se. However, there are recommended calorie levels that govern the number of servings you're allowed for every food group. So, you must select the proper levels and adjust periodically as your age changes. Nevertheless, you do not have to count or keep track of your calories.

However, to follow the Dash food regimen carefully, you will need to measure quantities and count the number servings of ingredients that fall into each food group. This is just as tedious if not more time consuming than calorie counting.

To begin with, this part of this system may be overwhelming for some people.

Not Specifically Designed for Weight Loss

The DASH food regimen does not include a fast weight loss phase (offered by most of the weight reduction diet options) in which the observers are able to lose weight relatively quickly which boosts motivation and encourages them to continue to follow the plan. Weight loss on the DASH Diet will be looked at specifically later in the book.

Not Appropriate for Everyone

Even though there are many people that can benefit from the DASH regimen, researchers have cautioned some groups of people to be careful as they adopt this eating plan.

A study was done to investigate the DASH Diet regimen in special populations. The researchers noted that while the food plan is healthy for most people, they noted that sufferers of chronic kidney disorder, persistent liver ailments, and people who are prescribed renin-angiotensin-aldosterone gadget antagonists must exercise caution. Additionally, they recommend that adjustments to the DASH weight loss program can be important for patients with chronic heart failure, out of control Type II diabetes, lactose intolerance, and celiac disease.

The report underscores the significance of working together with your healthcare provider before making significant modifications to your eating plan or fitness regimen. They may be able to refer you to a registered dietitian or another professional who can provide support and related services.

Estimating your needed calories

Data from the National Institute of Health states that a woman, aged 19-30, needs around 2000 calories per day if she is sedentary. If she is moderately active, she may need up to 2,200 calories per day. Active women will need up to 2,400 calories. For those aged 31-50, needed calories are about 200 per day lower in all categories.

For a sedentary man, aged 19-30, the daily caloric intake is 2,400 calories. A moderately active man will require between 2,600-2,800 calories, while an active man will need 3,000 calories per day. As men enter the age groups 31-50 and 51+, daily caloric needs for all categories drop about 200 calories per day.

Sedentary is defined as someone who only does light physical activity as part of their daily routine. In other words, they don't exercise. A moderately active person is defined as someone who engages in walking, maybe 1.5-3 miles per day. Active means a person who walks longer distances or who engages in more vigorous exercise such as running. However, your calorie needs are highly individual and determined by much more than your age and level of activity. You can look online for calorie calculators such as www.calculator.net/calorie-calculator.html to find out how many calories you need. This book does not focus on calorie counting as we think that focusing on eating a balanced diet is more beneficial for your health.

Recommended Servings for Different Food Groups in the DASH Diet

Given that the diet is rich in whole grains, vegetables, fruits, lean meat, and dairy products with low-fat content, this section aims at giving a general guide of the recommended servings that will help you adhere to the 2000 calories recommended in a day.

Grains Servings

Aim to have 6 six and 8 serving of grain per day. This includes cereal, bread, pasta, or rice. One serving consists of an ounce of dry cereal, a single slice of whole-wheat bread or half a cup of cooked rice, pasta, or cereal.

Whole grains are an excellent dietary choice. They are rich in nutrients and fiber when compared to refined grains. When grocery shopping, choose brown rice, whole-grain bread, and whole-wheat pasta. Always select products with the "100% whole grain" label. When preparing grains, avoid adding cheese, cream, or butter sauces. Grains naturally have low-fat content and they should be prepared in a way that maximizes this benefit.

Fruit Servings

The beauty of fresh fruit is that they require little to no time to prepare. They can be eaten as snacks or as part of a meal. Fruit, just like vegetables, are very rich in potassium, magnesium, and fiber. They also have low-fat content, with coconut being the only exception.

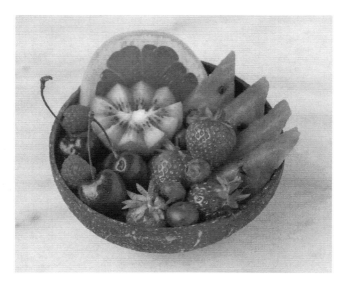

Picture source: unsplash.com

The DASH Diet recommended fruit servings are between 4 and 5 per day. A single serving can be one whole fruit or half a cup of frozen or canned fruit. Four ounces of a pure fruit juice is also equal to one serving.

You should strive to have at least a piece of fruit after every meal and another piece as a snack in between meals. A dessert of fresh fruit after an evening meal is a great way to round out your day. If you are consuming canned fruit or fruit juice, ensure that there is no added sugar. Ensure that juice is fresh fruit juice with no chemical additives.

Whenever possible, you should eat edible peels. Fruit such as apples, pears, and even mangoes have edible peels. These peels offer additional nutrients and fiber.

While fruit is generally recommended, you should be selective in the fruit you are consuming. Some fruit, especially citrus fruits and juices, may not be recommended if you are taking certain medications. If you are taking any medication, consult with your doctor regarding which types of fruit are recommended.

Vegetable Servings

Recommended servings for vegetables are between 4 and 5 servings per day. One cup of leafy vegetables (raw) or 1/2 cup of cut-up raw or cooked cut-up vegetables amounts to one serving.

The most common and recommended vegetables for the DASH Diet include carrots, tomatoes, greens, broccoli, and sweet potatoes. These vegetables are rich in minerals such as magnesium and potassium. They also have very high vitamin and fiber content.

Vegetables are an excellent dietary choice, given that they can be added to any meal. They can also be prepared as the main dish. When shopping for vegetables, choose the freshest ones. If you are buying canned or frozen vegetables, ensure that they have low sodium content.

Dairy Servings

The DASH Diet recommends 2 to 3 servings per day of dairy products. Milk, cheese, and yogurt are highly recommended as they are very rich in vitamin D, protein, and calcium. One of the key characteristics of the DASH Diet is low-fat content. When choosing dairy products to add to your meals, check the label to ensure that you are choosing a product with low-fat content.

A single dairy serving can be comprised of 1 cup of low-fat yogurt, skim, or milk. 1 ½ ounce of part-skim cheese also amounts to a single serving.

Frozen yogurt with low or no fat is a great way to boost the number of dairy products you consume. Yogurt also offers a sweet, but healthy treat,

Choose lactose-free products or an over-the-counter dairy product if you are lactose intolerant. In addition, go easy on the cheese as cheeses typically have high sodium levels.

Lean Meat, Fish, and Poultry Servings

If you are like most people, chances are that meat is one of the key components of your meals. Meat is rich in protein, zinc, iron, and B vitamins. In the DASH Diet, lean meat varieties are preferred. It is recommended that you have a maximum of 6 serving or less of lean meat in a week. An easy way to make your meal healthier is to cut back on the meat and add more vegetables. This is a healthier diet than having more meat and less vegetables.

In meat, fat is always concentrated under the skin. Trim away the skin and the fat from the meat before you prepare it. Instead of frying the meat, grill, roast, or boil it. This ensures that excess fat is removed. Fried meat will soak in more fat, increasing the fat content in your meal.

Fish such as herring, salmon, and tuna have high Omega-3 content which is helpful in lowering cholesterol levels.

Seeds, Legumes, and Nuts Servings

The recommended servings for seeds, nuts, and legumes are 4 to 5 in a week. These are good sources of protein, potassium, and magnesium. They also have high fiber and phytochemical levels which are helpful in protecting you against cardiovascular disease and some cancers.

The recommended servings are relatively small with the consumption limited to just a few times in a week. The reason for this is that these foods are rich in calories. A single serving is equivalent to 2 tablespoons of seeds, half a cup of cooked peas or beans, or a third cup of nuts.

When consuming nuts, add them to salads or cereals for a healthier meal. You can use seeds and legumes as an alternative if you do not eat meat. Soybean products are also good choices.

Sweets Servings

You can also incorporate sweets into your DASH Diet. if you are careful to limit your intake. The maximum servings you can have in a week is 5. A tablespoon of jelly, sugar or jam, 1 cup of lemonade, or ½ cup sorbet is equivalent to one serving.

The same dietary rules apply to sweets. Stick to sweets that are low in fat or those that have no fat at all. Sorbet, jelly beans, graham crackers, fruit ices, or low-fat cookies are great choices to consider. Avoid added sugar at all cost. It offers no nutritional value. You will only be adding to your calories.

Fats and Oils Servings

Fats help your body absorb and utilize essential vitamins. They also ensure that your immune system functions effectively. However, when in excess, fats can be quite harmful. Excess fats increase the chances of developing obesity, diabetes, or heart disease.

The DASH Diet ensures that you consume just the right amount of fats to keep your body healthy. 2 to 3 servings per day are recommended. 1 teaspoon of soft margarine, two tablespoons of salad dressing, or a tablespoon of mayonnaise amount to one serving.

Make sure to limit the consumption of foods that are rich in fats such as meat, cheese, whole milk, eggs, and butter, among others. You also should be cautious of trans-fat that is common in fried items, baked goods, and other processed foods.

You will have to adopt the new habit of always reading the labels of the products you are buying when doing your grocery shopping. Choose those that are free of trans-fat and those that have the lowest saturated fat.

DASH Diet Beverages

Here are some healthy options for drinks and beverages that can be included in the DASH Diet.

1. Water

This is an obvious one. It is at top of the list since it is the healthiest and perhaps the most readily available drink. It is recommended that a person consume eight glasses of water in a day. Since it can be difficult to attain the recommended number of glasses, you can compensate with fleshy fruits and vegetables because they have high water content. Another option is to make soup using foods such as meat and legumes.

The important thing is to ensure that you consume a lot of water daily.

2. Coffee

Another great low-calorie beverage is coffee. The best coffee is made with espresso and water only. This might sound a bit flat and you might think of making it better by adding some of your favorite ingredients. Don't. Get rid of your sweet tooth. The more the ingredients you add, the more calories you add in the coffee.

The transition to drinking plain coffee can be a bit challenging at first, but the more often you have it, the more you will get used to it. It is more beneficial to your health in the long run.

3. Tea

Tea is another good beverage choice if you are on a DASH Diet. Tea slows the rate of sugar intake in the body, hence regulating your blood sugar levels.

Hibiscus tea is one of the most effective beverages to have if you are on the DASH Diet. This tea contains anthocyanins an antioxidant that helps prevent blood vessels from narrowing. It is one of those "fast-action" beverages.

4. Smoothies

You can enjoy a DASH Diet smoothie. You can choose a turmeric smoothie, a skinny margarita, or a spicy Bloody Mary to accompany your meal.

5. Pomegranate Juice

Pomegranate juice has been proven to increase a person's systolic blood pressure. Its antioxidant content is three times that of green tea. It is an excellent beverage choice if you are on the DASH Diet.

Some Alcohol?

It has been proven that when you drink too much alcohol, chances of your blood pressure increasing shoot up drastically. With this knowledge, if you are on the DASH Diet, you should limit your alcohol consumption to the recommended levels. Women should stick to one drink or less per day. Men should limit alcohol consumption to two drinks or less in a day.

Chapter 3. How DASH is different from other popular diets

There are so many diets on the market. Let's have a look at some of the popular ones and how they compare with the DASH Diet

The Atkins Diet

The Atkins Diet is a low carb diet, so it's very different from the DASH Diet. Atkins advises followers to limit consumption of carbohydrates to 20 grams per day for the first few weeks, which is the "Induction Phase." This phase is designed to put your body in "ketosis" where you're burning fat rather than blood sugar for fuel. Over time, the restriction on carb consumption is relaxed, but following the Atkins Diet, you will never consume the level of carbohydrates you will on the DASH Diet. The Atkins Diet also puts no restrictions on sodium intake at all.

The Keto Diet

The Keto Diet is a version of the Atkins Diet or we should probably say that the other way around. The Keto Diet was developed many decades before the Atkins Diet. Originally it was developed to treat children with epilepsy. Like Atkins, it's designed to operate on the principle of "ketosis," so you burn fat rather than blood sugar for energy. It also proposes a similar radical restriction of carbohydrate consumption, but unlike Atkins does so for the long haul. If you follow the Keto Diet, you will limit your carbohydrate intake to 20 grams per day or less for life. Unlike Atkins, Keto also restricts protein intake to about 15-30% of total calories. The Keto Diet makes no restriction on the amount of salt consumed; in fact, some Keto experts advise consuming more salt.

The Paleo Diet

The "Paleo" Diet or as it's sometimes called the "Primal" Diet" is based on the belief that primitive humans consumed certain foods (during the Paleolithic era) and that our bodies are designed to eat these foods. Whether their compiled list of foods is accurate or not is up for interpretation, but basically, you can think of Paleo as Atkins with some add-ons that will up your carbohydrate intake, but without consuming any processed or modern varieties. For example, sweet potato is acceptable on Paleo, but bread and pasta are not since they are foods invented by civilized man. While you can consume more carbs (or limit them), there are no specific rules for consuming fat and protein and adherents often like to consume more fatty goods for energy. They also strongly advise eating grass-fed beef as opposed to standard beef, which is grain-fed. Like the other diets mentioned, salt is not restricted.

The South Beach Diet

The South Beach Diet was a very popular diet in the late 1990s, but appears to have lost steam, being wiped out by Paleo and Keto in the Diet Wars. The South Beach Diet was a knock off of the Atkins Diet and not much more than a marketing ploy. It can be thought of as a modernized version of Atkins in the sense that at the time the South Beach Diet was developed, leaner meats were favored as that was in the middle of the "fat is bad" era. The South Beach Diet promoted low carb eating, but with lean cuts of meat.

The Mediterranean Diet

Like the DASH Diet, the Mediterranean Diet has gained a widespread following among medical and health professionals. However, as we reviewed earlier, the DASH Diet was created by doctors who were doing research trying to treat blood pressure using diet. The Mediterranean Diet, in contrast, was not invented by anyone; it's simply the way that people in the Mediterranean basin eat and have been eating for countless centuries. It's not all that different from the DASH Diet, except that it does not restrict salt and it encourages the consumption of some red wine. The Mediterranean Diet also emphasizes the consumption of fatty fish, such as mackerel and sardines, varieties which are readily available in the Mediterranean Sea. It encourages liberal use of olive oil and consumption of nuts which contrasts with the restrictions on oil use and nuts in the DASH Diet. However, the similarities between the two diets are strong enough that some nutritionists have been pushing a combination of the two diets called the "DASH Mediterranean Solution".

Readers may be interested in looking into the DASH Mediterranean Solution, so let's take some time to review the foods typical of the Mediterranean Diet. Keep in mind that the food pyramid isn't anything official because this is nothing more than the native diet consumed in Greece, Israel, coastal Italy, southern France, Morocco, and of course Spain and Portugal, which are probably the two best representatives of the Mediterranean Diet.

Based on the eating patterns of people in these regions, the nutritional community has concocted a food pyramid. At its base are whole grains, including bread, rice, and pasta, among others. Unlike the DASH Diet, the Mediterranean Diet doesn't offer specific guidance on serving sizes or number of servings per day, only relative servings between different food groups. Beans and nuts are often included with whole grains at the bottom of the pyramid.

Next, you're advised to eat large amounts of fruits and vegetables. On the next level of the pyramid, we find olive oil. This is a major distinction between the DASH Diet – which severely limits oil intake, even healthy oils – and the Mediterranean Diet. On the Mediterranean Diet, you're advised to consume olive oil in large amounts. You can also consume related oils (those based on monounsaturated fat) such as avocado oil.

The only recommendations for the lower three levels of the Mediterranean Diet pyramid are that you consume them "daily" and that you have mostly whole grains, then fruits and vegetables in slightly lower amounts, and olive oil in slightly lower amounts.

Above this, we have fish and seafood. According to those advising this diet plan, you should consume fish and seafood "a few times a week," but we imagine if you lived on the southern coast of Spain or Italy, you might be eating more seafood than that. In addition to eating fatty varieties of mackerel, sardines, and anchovies, you can eat lean seafood like octopus, squid, and scallops.

49

The next category is eggs, cheese, poultry, and yogurt. The only advice given here is to consume them "daily to weekly." For cheese and yogurt, there is not any specification as to whether to consume low-fat or regular varieties. We suspect that in traditional cultures regular, whole-fat varieties were consumed. There are no specifications to eat skinless poultry.

Finally, at the top of the pyramid, we have meats and sweets. By meats, in this case, they mean red meat and pork, and probably lamb, which is very popular throughout the region. There are no restrictions on fat in the meat. However, you should be consuming "meats" in small amounts or weekly. Whether anyone living in the area follows the rules this closely is up for debate, of course.

So now that you know what the Mediterranean diet is, how would you go about combining it with the DASH Diet? Start with the Mediterranean Diet and simply limit sodium intake to 2,300 mg per day. Second, you can follow the portion guidelines advised in the DASH Diet, along with with the servings per day guidelines.

With these minor adjustments to the Mediterranean Diet to align more with the DASH Diet, you should experience positive health benefits from following this plan. If you're not getting results, you could cut back on olive oil (which may be healthy, but being fat, it is packed with calories) and make other adjustments, such as eating skinless chicken.

Dash Diet in the Global Diet Rankings

A study to rank the best 40 diets has been undertaken by the U.S News and World Report, beginning in 2001. The ranking looks at different aspects of the diets to determine which diet plans are most effective. This study has ranked the DASH Diet as the best overall diet plan according to very strict criteria (easy to follow, nutritious, safe, effective for short & long-term weight loss, helps fight diabetes & heart disease) for eight consecutive years that the ranking has been undertaken (2001 – 2018).

It has been reliably proven that the DASH Diet is as effective or even better at lowering blood pressure levels prescription medications.

The diet has also been proven to reduce symptoms of hypertension in research that was funded by the NIH Heart, Lung and Blood Institute (NHLB) when they developed the diet.

The consistent high rankings of the diet over the years has led to it being recommended for the general public by many health professionals. Janet de Jesus, from NHLBI's Center for Translation Research and Implementation Science, states that the importance of the DASH Diet combined with the reduced-sodium intake has a significant impact on general health, including lowering blood pressure.

Research by the same NHLBI had also shown that those who adopted the DASH Diet saw a significant reduction in blood pressure levers within a few weeks. Reduced blood pressure reduces the chances of heart-related diseases such as hypertension.

Advantages of the DASH Diet compared to other diets

Except for the Mediterranean Diet, the DASH Diet offers several key advantages:

Unlike complicated point-counting schemes, the DASH Diet is quite easy to follow. Portioning out your servings is a snap.

• The DASH Diet can be described as a careful application of "normal eating," so you're never going to feel deprived.

• The focus on limiting sodium and balancing sodium, potassium, magnesium, and calcium on the DASH Diet makes it great for promoting cardiovascular health.

• Unlike radical diets such as Atkins or Keto, it doesn't require you to give up entire food groups for the rest of your life.

• Unlike Paleo, it's not based on a made-up fad.

Chapter 4. The DASH Diet and Weight Loss

Normally people come to a diet hoping to achieve weight loss and they consider health benefits such as those we have discussed as a nice side benefit. The DASH Diet often attracts people because they have been diagnosed with high blood pressure and their doctor has advised them to seek out the kind of lifestyle changes that the DASH Diet offers. Regardless of the reasons why you came to the DASH Diet, it can lead to substantial weight loss.

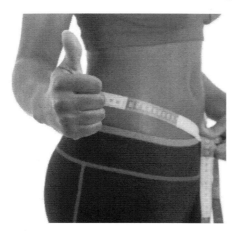

Picture source: nutritionfacts.org

Since the diet focuses on eating the right foods with the right portions, it's also effective for short- and long-term weight loss.

Effortless Weight Loss

The DASH Diet isn't all that difficult to follow because in many cases, it simply mirrors what people normally eat already, with a few adjustments. Instead of eating barbecued pork ribs, you eat a skinless barbecued chicken breast. You can have potato salad but use low-fat mayo. Adjustments like these aren't all that difficult when compared to following a Keto or Atkins Diet, where you can't consume either barbecue sauce or eat potatoes.

Portion Control

Some diets use complicated systems for portion control. Most people don't want to mix accounting with eating, so while these diets may still attract some people, most people will find it to be too much trouble in the long run.

Other diets which fall into the low-fat category are based largely on counting calories. These types of diets can leave you feeling hungry and irritable. You may grow tired and mentally foggy since your body isn't getting enough to get by and you're not feeling full.

The DASH Diet avoids calorie counting altogether. Instead, you simply follow the rules for the portion sizes outlined earlier and then eat the number of items that the DASH food pyramid advises, Provided you're not overindulging, it is quite simple to follow.

By specifying the maximum number of portions, you can eat each day from each food group, you automatically get portion control without having to count calories or follow a complicated system. With an emphasis on low-calorie fruits and veggies and the consumption of a lot of fiber, you will also find that you will feel full. You won't feel deprived, even though you're limiting portion sizes and numbers of portions consumed daily.

Limited Meat Consumption

We aren't advocating that people become vegan or vegetarian, although that is an option if you want to pursue it. One benefit of following the DASH Diet is that it limits meat consumption. In American society, people eat meat without any regard to portion size or even how many times per day they are eating it. Many people eat some kind of meat item for breakfast, lunch, and dinner. They might even snack on it.

The DASH Diet forces you to think about how much meat you're eating, maybe for the very first time in your life. It also restricts servings of meat to not more than 6 servings per week. That's a very easy rule to follow and if you are following it for the first time, you're going to be reducing the overall level of calories consumed per day significantly.

By cutting off the fat on beef and pork and skin on poultry, another source of calories can be eliminated. This will contribute to weight loss if you haven't been paying much attention to unnecessary fat on meat.

Eat Those Fruits and Veggies

What is the main benefit of eating several servings of spinach per day? Well, spinach is packed with all kinds of cancer-fighting nutrients and contains important minerals such as potassium, but the advantage we're looking for here is that spinach is very low calorie. You can eat a lot of spinach, broccoli, cauliflower, and other veggies and fill yourself up without consuming large amounts of calories. The high fiber in the fruits and vegetables will help you feel satiated faster and reduce the temptation to eat unnecessary meats and oils. The result will be more weight loss.

Regulating Sweets

The DASH Diet will help you get a handle on sweets and desserts – provided that you're truly committed to the diet, of course. First, the DASH Diet tells you exactly how many servings to eat –

five per week. Second, it has strict definitions of what counts as a "sweet" with the size of each serving specified in detail. Sure – you could cheat if you wanted – but then don't blame anyone else if you fail to reach your health and weight loss goals. However, if you follow the rules, you will find the fact that the DASH Diet allows some sweets will help you satisfy that old sweet tooth and secondly, that you will be losing weight, despite consuming five servings of sweets per week.

Final Thoughts

The DASH Diet does not make a pie in the sky promises about weight loss. Keto, Atkins, and many other diets do make such claims. The DASH Diet takes an entirely different approach, more akin to the turtle that wins the race than the hare, who has a good start in the race but loses.

The DASH Diet will generate slow, but steady weight loss that will add up over time provided that you follow the rules. Once you fully adjust to the rules to be followed on a diet, you will find that it gets easier to follow as time goes on. When people get tired of avoiding pasta for the rest of their lives and cheat on their deprivation diets, you'll still be following yours since it's not much different from what people would eat already. The DASH Diet is just a healthier version of a typical diet with the relative proportions of foods changed around to promote more consumption of potassium and magnesium.

So the takeaways are:

• The DASH Diet will help you lose weight.

• Expect weight loss to be gradual and slow, but steady. Don't look to lose 20 pounds in 10 days.

• The DASH Diet is not a quick fix for weight loss – it's a lifestyle plan developed for overall health.

• The DASH Diet won't just help you lose weight; it will help you keep your blood pressure under control as you age (and reduce it if you've developed hypertension) and avoid diabetes as well as many other health problems.

Chapter 5. Transitioning to the DASH Diet

You've decided to transition to a DASH Diet. You already know its benefits, but where do you begin? Worry no more. I am about to give you steps to assist you in transitioning to a DASH Diet correctly. The hardest part of a journey is taking the first step. When you look back, you'll be amazed at just how much you've achieved. This is because the DASH Diet is not rocket science and getting the ingredients and preparing the meals is pretty easy. The good thing about it is that you are not completely throwing away your typical eating plan, but you are incorporating the DASH Diet principles into how you eat. Some days you'll feel like eating more and other days less for a particular food category. That's okay, as long as you don't steer too much from the recommendations. The only thing that doctors give as an exception is sodium. It is highly advisable not to exceed the limit for sodium.

As you get started on the DASH Diet, you will need to unlearn some of these misconceptions about the diet as well as educate those around you about the benefits of your new eating plan. This will go a long way in having people to support you and hold you accountable along the way.

• The DASH Diet is only for individuals with high blood pressure - while the diet helps individuals that have high blood pressure, they are not the only ones who need to be concerned with what they are taking into their bodies. Exceeding the limits of recommended sodium intake can take a toll on anyone's body.

• The sole focus of a DASH Diet is low sodium or no salt - sodium reduction is a recommendation, but not the only one. Other nutrients which play a role in good health are recommended.

• The DASH Diet is an "all or nothing diet"- this is a common misconception that prevents people from transitioning to a DASH Diet. Many people are reluctant to start the plan for fear of failing and having side effects after returning to old eating habits. The diet is all about incorporating better food choices into your meal plans in ways that are realistic and achievable.

Let's look at an overall plan to consider when transitioning to the DASH Diet.

These are the things you want to eat more of:

• Nuts
• Fruits
• Low-fat or Fat-Free Dairy

- Whole grains
- Vegetables
- Lean Meat, Fish, and Poultry.

Foods that you will eat less of or totally eliminate:

- Sodium
- Fatty meats
- Saturated and Trans Fats
- Sugar and Sweets

Keep in mind that you don't want to transition to the diet all at once. As you introduce new foods, especially those rich in fiber, your digestion may change. You'll want to slowly and gradually incorporate them into your meal plans until it becomes a routine. The changes could be over a couple of days or even weeks. As the DASH Diet has high fiber, fluid intake should be increased at the same time. Fiber tends to draw water into the bowel, which could lead to hard stool and constipation.

As you begin the DASH Diet, clean out your cupboards, removing those sugary, salty foods and snacks that might tempt you in the future. Donate the food to a local food bank.

Another important thing to note is that on the DASH Diet, you will limit the number of times that you eat out. The quantities of sugar, fats, and oils contained in restaurant foods are almost impossible to know.

5 Steps to Note While Transitioning to the DASH Diet

1. Maintain a food diary

This could be an app or a physical diary. This diary is where you will record the changes you see.   It is also a place to set daily nutritional goals. This will give you a sense of accountability and can also be used if there is a need to see a doctor.

2. Do not skip meals

The DASH Diet includes a minimum of three meals. Don't skip lunch and then say you'll make up for it in the evening.

3. Be cautious with food labels

You are focusing on reducing sodium in this diet. When shopping, read labels. If a label says "reduced sodium," run for your life. Reduced sodium does not mean its low. A low sodium diet has 140mg of sodium per serving. The recommended daily sodium intake per day is less than 2,300 mg.

4. Compare DASH with your current meal plan

Depending on your eating patterns, choose to either increase or decrease your food portions.

5. Begin the DASH Diet

Being equipped with information about the DASH Diet is not enough. Start working on it. The key is to plan and stock your kitchen with the recommended DASH foods. Based on your eating preferences, create a meal plan to help you make better decisions when you are shopping.

Creating a Meal Plan

The meal plan should be made with the following eating times in mind at a minimum.

1. Breakfast

2. Lunch

3. Dinner.

Keep the following in mind while and before shopping.

1. Don't shop when hungry - You know those foods, especially fast food and the sugary foods that you can't resist eating? Well, the desire to eat them is very high when hungry. Eat before you go shopping.

2. Read food labels - for packaged food, read their nutrition labels. Be extra aware of the fat and sodium content as earlier stated.

3. Less packaged and fresher food - Instead of going for canned fruits, choose the fresh ones. The same rule applies to vegetables. Fresh foods, in most cases still have their original nutrients and therefore have more health benefits.

Breakfast options

As earlier stated, the DASH Diet doesn't have a specific list of food to eat. The focus is on serving different food groups at each meal. The following breakfast shopping list will enable you to try different DASH breakfast recipe meals.

- Whole-wheat bread
- Eggs
- Bananas
- Low-fat milk
- Oatmeal
- Peanut butter
- Yogurt

- Cranberry juice
- Trans-free margarine
- Skim milk
- Strawberries or raspberries

Lunch list

- Green vegetables such as spinach, kale, broccoli
- Almonds
- Carrots
- Fruits such as melons, apricots, dates, grapes, mangoes, tangerines, and blueberries
- Turkey
- Whole-grain crackers

Dinner

- Olive oil
- Whole wheat spaghetti
- Beef
- Wild rice
- Chicken
- Tuna
- Broccoli
- Potatoes
- Green peas

Narrowing down to the individual food groups

Whole grains- sources of whole grains include whole-grain bread, whole-grain cereals, brown rice, oatmeal

Vegetables - vegetables can go up to 5 servings per day. This includes leafy green vegetables such as kale and spinach. Other recommended vegetables include broccoli, carrots, tomatoes, Brussels sprouts, and sweet potatoes. They are packed with high fiber, potassium, magnesium, and healthy vitamins. Both raw and cooked vegetables work well. Avoid frozen vegetables.

Fruits- also up to 5 serving per day. The DASH Diet includes eating a lot of fruit. Recommended fruits are apples, pineapples, grapes, berries, peaches, and mangoes. It is highly recommended that you eat edible peels of fruit such as apples and pears. The peels contain healthy nutrients and fiber. Fruit can be enjoyed as a side dish with other meals or as a snack. If you have to buy canned fruit, check the label for added sugar which should be avoided. Fruit such as grapefruit can clash with certain medications, so it is advisable to consult your doctor or a pharmacist before their use.

Dairy Products - could be up to 3 servings per day. Dairy products in the DASH Diet should have low fat: low-fat cheese, low-fat yogurt, and skim milk. Consult with your doctor if you are lactose intolerant or have a hard time digesting dairy. They will most probably describe pills that can aid in digestion and reduce the effects of dairy intolerance.

Fish, Meat, and Lean Chicken - 6 or fewer helpings per day. Be keen to reduce red meat and increase white meat. Tuna and salmon have omega-3 fatty acids, which lower cholesterol. What does one serving of meat look like? The size of your palm is a good guide: an average palm estimate is 3 ounces. Avoid fatty meat such as bacon. Also, remove the fat and skin from poultry and meat. If possible, bake, grill, or broil meat instead of frying.

Legumes, seeds, grains, and nuts - these include walnuts, peanuts, peas, lentils, rice, pasta, sunflower seeds, and kidney beans. It is recommended that you have up to 4 or 5 servings per week. The serving size for these foods is rather small because they contain high-fat content and a lot of calories.

Look for whole-grain bread which has more nutrients compared to refined grains. Be on the lookout for products labeled "100 percent whole wheat'. Also, learn to enjoy grains without adding things such as butter or cheese which have fat. For a nice crunch, you can try sprinkling them on salads. Soybean-based products are good alternatives to meat because just like meat, they contain all amino acids required by the body to make a complete protein.

Oils and fats (2-3 servings per day) – choosing the right oil is important. Too much fat increases one's chances of heart disease, diabetes, and obesity. Just to clarify, fat is not necessarily a bad thing; it helps your immune system. The key thing is to avoid trans fats in fried and processed foods. Saturated fat is also a key culprit in increasing the risk of coronary artery disease. The DASH Diet highly recommends vegetable oils: corn oil, olive oil, and canola oil. Read labels on things such as margarine to select those that are trans-fat-free and that have low amounts of saturated fats.

Sugar - cutting all sugar out of your diet all at once might be a difficult task. The alternative is to use things such as honey, agave syrup, and maple syrup in extremely limited quantities. You can sneak something like a diet cola into your meals, but it should not be a substitute for plain water. Cut back on added sugar which only adds calories and has no nutritional value.

Sweets - up to 5 servings or fewer a week is permitted. The DASH Diet is not harsh; it doesn't require that you banish sweets all at once. It advises you to go easy on them by choosing those that are fat-free or low fat.

The suggestions above are just to get you started on the DASH Diet and they are not the only foods permitted, but it's wise to use the following guidelines and tips:

• Reduce or limit the intake of sugary foods and beverages.
• Use vegetable oils for cooking
• More white meat, less red meat
• Low-fat or fat-free dairy products
• Be careful and observant with sodium on food labels
• Measure fresh fruit juice portions
• Drink alcohol sparingly and coffee in moderation. The recommended amount of alcohol for women is a maximum of 1 drink per day or less and for men is a maximum of 2 drinks per day or less
• Use herbs and spices to enhance flavor instead of adding salt
• If you have to buy canned food, rinse food such as beans to wash away excess salt
• You can substitute sugar with honey or other natural sweeteners in baking or beverages
• Serve fruit as snacks

- Reduce salad dressing

If you have existing medical conditions, it is wise to see a doctor who will help you in developing a personalized DASH Diet to best meet your overall health needs.

Incorporating Physical Exercise to the DASH Diet

Exercising in conjunction with the DASH Diet will yield even more benefits. Exercising on its own has its benefits. Imagine the benefits of combining a good exercise program with the DASH Diet. The DASH Diet in all its moderation will not require you to do high-intensity exercises. Do something you enjoy at a moderate activity level.

Some of the moderate activities you could include are cycling, walking, swimming, house chores, and light aerobics.

The recommended amount of exercise is at least 2hrs and 30 minutes per week of activity at a moderate intensity. Gradually increase to 5 hours per week. More on fitness will be covered in a later chapter.

Set Up Your Kitchen

Just as you need to select the ingredients you know you will use, select kitchen equipment you are comfortable with. The recipes in this book require a minimum amount of equipment, while still taking advantage of labor-saving devices. Make your kitchen a friendly, welcoming, organized place. Your time in the kitchen should be pleasant and it should be easy for you to prep and prepare meals. The following two lists include essential equipment and nice-to-have equipment.

Essential Equipment

This list of essential equipment includes items needed for daily cooking, aimed at the beginner cook:

Nonstick skillet or frying pan with lid.

A good nonstick skillet is indispensable, making it easy to brown, fry, and sauté. Choose a size that works for you, considering the number of people in your household.

A small and a large pot, with lids.

A small and a large saucepan will be used in this book to prepare sauces, soups, and stews. Choosing ones with a nonstick coating will make clean up easy and won't require a lot of oil when using. Nontoxic eco-friendly options include glass, ceramic, stainless steel, and green nonstick cookware.

Baking dishes.

Glass or metal baking dishes are used for roasting meats and preparing casserole-type dishes. They are even useful for serving straight from the oven to the table and can be used to store leftovers.

Rimmed 9-by-13-inch baking sheet.

A baking sheet with a 1-inch rim is designed to catch juices from roasting vegetables, meats, fish, and poultry. Choose from metal or silicone.

Knives.

The two most important knives for efficient prep in the kitchen are a good-quality chef's knife for larger items such as meats and a paring knife for fruit, vegetables, and herbs.

Cutting boards.

A wooden cutting board will be easy on kitchen knives, keeping them sharp for longer. Dedicated cutting boards are ideal—one for fresh fruits and vegetables, one for meats—but this isn't always practical on a tight budget. If you are using one cutting board, be sure to avoid cross-contamination by sanitizing your board after working with raw meats and seafood.

Assorted mixing bowls.

Look for durable nesting bowls that can handle large and small volumes. Look for bowls with lids, which can be used for storing leftovers.

Blender.

A basic blender is needed to make smoothies and can also take the place of a food processor for puréeing soups and beans. Try to purchase one with at least 450 watts of power so you have the flexibility needed to effortlessly process a variety of ingredients.

Other tools. Other kitchen necessities you should have on hand include a slotted spoon, spatula, wooden spoon, whisk, ladle, can opener, colander, measuring cups and spoons, timer, meat thermometer, vegetable peeler, oven mitts, pot holder and kitchen towels.

Nice-to-Have Equipment

Food processor.

A food processor is nice to have for chopping, slicing, grating, dicing, and puréeing a variety of ingredients including nuts, beans, soups, vegetables, and grains. Food processors are similar to blenders, but they have interchangeable blades and discs rather than a fixed blade.

Spiralizer.

A spiralizer turns fresh veggies into faux noodles. Most models are about the size of a large toaster and function like a giant pencil sharpener. Spiralizing veggies and using them in place of pasta is a great way to boost your intake of vegetables while cutting back on calories.

Slow cooker.

A slow cooker has many advantages and is a great way to save time while preparing a nutritious meal. Slow cookers can be used for breakfast casseroles, steel-cut oats, soups, stews, roasts, and grains.

Chapter 6. Physical Exercises and Dash Diet

Exercise is an important component of your health regimen. However, it's important to recognize that for many of us, exercise is not going to lead to significant weight loss. The bottom line is that to achieve weight loss from exercise; you'd have to spend a significant amount of time engaged in physical activity each day and train at a high level. Many of us don't have the time for that and diet is far more effective than exercise when it comes to weight loss.

When you engage in a cardiovascular exercise, which is extremely strenuous, you can even scar the heart and raise the body's level of inflammation. It's hard to believe, but it's true – people who engage in high-intensity exercise are actually at elevated risk of a heart attack. It seems paradoxical until you realize that a heart attack can also be caused by increased inflammation.

For these reasons, the DASH dieter should focus on moderate exercise. The definition of moderate exercise is not entirely rigorous. However, remember that you're not exercising to lose weight — instead, the DASH dieter exercises to maintain general good health.

That said, when it comes to blood pressure, as we'll see in a moment, the effects of the DASH Diet are enhanced by regular aerobic exercise.

Benefits of Aerobic Exercise

We'll investigate the different options that are available when it comes to exercise in a moment. For now, let's examine some of the health benefits.

Exercise lowers the overall risk of death. The risk of death decreases for all causes – indicating that exercise reduces the risk of death from cancer, cardiovascular disease, kidney disease, and possibly many others.

Regular exercise will help you maintain healthy blood levels. Even if you already have hypertension, you should get out there and get moving so that your health problems don't get any worse. Exercise may help some mildly hypertensive patients by widening your blood vessels as they need to carry extra blood to the large muscle groups to keep them adequately supplied during physical activity. This helps your blood vessels stay in shape, remaining supple and pliant, rather than stiff and brittle. That means they will better respond to changes in blood pressure and stress.

Aerobic exercise can raise your HDL (high-density lipoprotein cholesterol) level and lower LDL (low-density lipoprotein cholesterol) cholesterol. By engaging in regular aerobic exercise, you can lower the chances of acquiring heart disease by improving your blood lipids.

In addition to benefits that affect blood lipids, exercise will strengthen your heart. Why? Because when you're engaged in physical activity, your blood pressure goes up and the heart has to work harder to pump blood. Just like any muscle, when the heart has to work hard, it gets stronger. When your heart is stronger, it won't need to beat as much.

One of the benefits of regular exercise is that it will help you stay independent as you get older. By helping maintaining balance and muscle strength, you can avoid having to get around using a walker, or worse, ending up in a nursing home before your time.

Exercise can also help you maintain healthy blood sugar levels. The more conditioned your large muscles are, the better they're going to be at using and metabolizing blood sugar appropriately. For this reason, your doctor may suggest you start an exercise program if you become pre-diabetic.

Another benefit of exercise is that it can improve your mood. This won't come as a shock to those who already exercise, but for those who are not used to tying up their running shoes, they may not be aware of the endorphin rush that you get while engaging in strenuous physical activity. Exercise is a great antidote to depression.

Does Exercise have to be intense?

The good news is that it doesn't. While you may believe that to get in shape, you've got to tie up your running shoes and run for five miles, research has shown that in fact, you get most of the benefit in the first few minutes of exercise, meaning that running for long periods of time isn't necessary. Alternatively, exercise research has also shown that moderate exercise provides almost as many benefits. Please note that the more moderate the exercise, the more time you should put into it. So, if you're planning on a walking program, you'll probably want to walk for about 30 minutes a day, five days a week. If you're hiking on steep mountain trails, you may need less exercise to achieve the same level of fitness. This also applies to running. Some recent research has shown that people who exercise at a high intensity but only do it for 1-5 minutes get the same benefit they would have gotten if they spent 20 minutes or a half-hour engaged in exercise. The key isn't really to obsess over what kind of exercise "works" and what doesn't as the reality is that any kind of exercise works. The key is to find something that you like doing and will stick to for the long term.

What Does the Science Say?

When it comes to the DASH Diet, the focus is on high blood pressure. So, we might ask, does the DASH Diet produce better results when combined with exercise? This question was asked by James Blumenthal and his colleagues in a study which compared obese subjects who followed the DASH Diet and exercised with obese subjects who followed the DASH Diet, but who did not exercise. The subjects of the study were either pre-hypertensive or had stage 1 high blood pressure. They found that DASH Diet subjects that also exercised reduced their systolic blood pressure more than 44% when compared with those who were on the DASH Diet alone. Diastolic blood pressure was also better for the DASH dieters who exercised, versus those who did not, although the results were not as dramatic.

This result is very important so let's state the conclusion again – people who follow the DASH Diet together with exercise end up with better blood pressure numbers than people who follow the DASH Diet alone. This does not mean everyone on the DASH Diet needs to exercise, although there are lots of reasons why everyone should exercise –the research does confirm that exercise is at least an option that you will want to consider.

Improved Cognitive Function

One of the benefits of the DASH Diet is it improves mental clarity and cognitive function. The DASH Diet alone, without any exercise, can reduce the risk of developing dementia and Alzheimer's disease. The reason for this is that high blood pressure increases the risk of these dreaded diseases, and by reducing blood sugar, the risk of getting dementia is reduced.

However, when people engage in exercise and follow the DASH Diet, it's been found that they have more mental focus and perform better on cognitive tests than do sedentary people.

Dash Diet is more effective when it is followed by exercise after a meal rather than just focusing on the meal plan. There are a few easy and comfortable forms of exercises you can include for effective weight loss.

Running

Running helps to improve the physical and mental health of a person. Running is very effective for all ages and health fitness levels. Did you know that running can reduce knee pain? Many overweight people suffer from knee pain caused by swollen knees. Running can have a significant impact on reducing knee pain. Running increases weight loss, whether it is outdoor running or treadmill running as it helps to burn calories. Those suffering from depression will find that running helps to improve their mood even after being stressed as it leads to a release of endorphins.

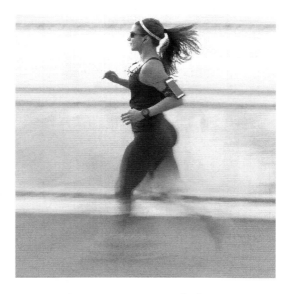

Picture source: unsplash.com

Hikes

Hiking is often considered a recreational activity, but it also has significant health benefits. According to various researchers, hiking has a positive impact on weight loss and overall health maintenance. It helps in reducing problems associated with heart disease and improves blood pressure levels, as well as improving body balance and muscle tone.

Swimming

Swimming is a great sport for improving general health as it requires people to use all parts of their body. Swimming improves muscle tone and strengthens the heart, as well as improving circulation. Swimming can contribute to weight loss as well as being an excellent way of relaxing.

Housework

Housework activities are a very important exercise for weight loss and the body. Housework not only burns calories through the efforts needed but also help to reduce stress. By engaging in these activities, the mind is distracted from the stressors in life.

Activities such as these are important and can bring a great change in people; these suggested activities are probably the best ones for beginners.

Thus change is impeccable. For beginners, I would recommend to follow these tips closely and observe every change that happens to them. Some are advised to reduce the amount of salt intake in the body, which is good, though excessive reduction of salt intake by itself is a danger as it impacts blood pressure.

Lifting Weights

Apart from the outdoor types of exercise, there are also indoor activities which are very effective for weight loss. If monitored well with a regular routine, they can add to the results brought by dietary changes. When it comes to exercise, it is important to start new types of exercise slowly. Before using weights, you should do basic exercises first to gradually prepare your body for heavier lifting.

Basics before Lifting Weights

Squats

Squats increase strength in muscles attached to the hips. Squats are simply done by squatting down and getting up. Squats prepare the legs for heavy lifts such as the deadlift which require a lot of energy from the legs.

Pull-ups and push-ups

This is another basic exercise to increase strength in the biceps and triceps muscles. Start by doing a few and then gradually increase the number of repetitions that you do.

Treadmill

This is an indoor activity that involves running or jogging on a moving track. Running on a treadmill can burn a significant amount of calories in a short time. The advantage of running on a treadmill is the fact that you can set the speed you want to run. For beginners, it is advised to start with low speed and then gradually increase the speed and incline.

How to Start Weightlifting for Beginners

Weightlifting used to be thought of as a suitable type of exercise for men as it was often geared towards building muscle mass. Weights are not just effective for increasing muscle mass, but for improving muscle tone and reducing weight in both men and women.

Most people who are new to exercising find it overwhelming when they enter a gym for the first time as they don't know where to start.

Here are some few tips to consider first before beginning on a weight program:

- Know how each weight is to be used before you use it
- Begin with a light weight until you learn the exercise
- Ask the gym staff about anything you are not sure of before you use it

Why is there no change after going to the gym?

This question is frequently asked by beginners to an exercise program. Everything requires time and commitment, and most importantly, patience. As a beginner, don't expect massive changes in your body after going to the gym for a short time. At times, you might not see any change yourself, but those around you may notice the changes brought on by exercise.

Below is a list of reasons why you may not see a significant change in your weight after hitting the gym for a month:

- Lifting weights that are too light
- Not using time effectively at the gym
- Doing the lifts the wrong way
- Not going to the gym consistently
- Not changing your workout routine regularly
- The wrong meal plan
- Eating a lot of calories before the gym

Chapter 7. DASH Diet FAQS

Can I still adopt the DASH Diet even if I don't have high blood pressure?

Yes, you can! By itself, the diet has benefits for anyone who wants to live a healthy lifestyle. Although the diet was originally formulated for those with high blood pressure, its focus on healthy foods makes it a good option even if you don't have high blood pressure.

Why should I use the DASH Diet instead of other diets on the market?

It is understandable to be skeptical about the diet. There is just way too much information out there that it's become hard to pick out what's the real deal and what isn't. You have people who are non-experts in health talking about this or that diet – yet they have no personal experience with it. The DASH Diet has gone through clinical trials with large samples of people and all with tremendous results. People are seeking answers for better ways to achieve the best versions of themselves. With the barrage of information coming at them, it's hard to see which path to take. In the end, for you to be sure, check in with your doctor and nutritionist for advice on whether or not the DASH Diet is worth trying.

When should I expect to see some significant results?

If you are vigilant in following the plan, you can expect to see results within a few weeks. If continue to consistently follow the DASH Diet, you will experience long-term weight loss.

What are my drinking options while on the DASH diet?

Low caloric drinks are most suitable for the DASH Diet. That makes water a perfect beverage to drink as part of this diet. Sugar-free juices and drinks are also a good option while on this diet.

Can I still have caffeine? And what about alcohol?

Caffeine and alcohol are permitted as part of the DASH Diet, but consumption is limited. Combine caffeine intake with a meal. Alcohol should be consumed sparingly with a limit of two alcoholic beverages per day for males and one per day for females.

How long should a person stay on this diet?

There are many significant health benefits to be gained by using this eating plan. It's better to make this plan a lifestyle rather than just adopting it for a few days or months. It an advisable to have the mindset and mentality that this is a permanent eating plan. Since the DASH Diet will not harm you in the long run, it is up to you and your health professional to make the decision as to how long you should follow this diet plan.

Why is Sodium such a big deal in the diet?

As this diet was originally developed to address issues of hypertension in patients, it focuses on reducing sodium intake to lower blood pressure.

Can you take medication while on this diet?

Some medication such as blood thinners can react with certain foods. It is always important to consult with your doctor or health practitioner before beginning a diet such as the DASH Diet.

If I feel sick while on this diet, should I discontinue it?

If you feel unwell while on this diet, you should consult with your health practitioner.

Can we use the diet while on medications?

It is not advised to switch to this diet while on any medication as it can interact with the diet routine and the foods included in the diet. Ask for a doctor's or health expert's advice as to whether you should continue the medications while you are on the diet or if you stop using them.

Is the diet still for me is if I am not a fan of fruit and not a vegetarian

Would you be willing to open your mind to fruit and veggies if I told you that people who don't eat enough of those foods are the ones who battle the most with their weight? If you want results, at least give this a try. You really have nothing to lose and just might find that you'll come to love fruits and veggies. There are ways to spruce up your meals, and this book will give you a fantastic meal plan to work with. A diet that's rich in fruits and veggies will help you lose the weight that you want.

How do I deal with my bad attitude towards fruits and vegetables

First of all, make a list before you go grocery shopping. Make it a plan to try out every vegetable that is available. This way, you can find out which ones are your favorite. Give it enough time and you'll be craving them!

A way to get more veggies into your diet is incorporating them into meals such as your morning omelet. Need a way to get the fruit in? Add them to your cereal. Make a habit of packing fruits and veggies with you when you head out to work or wherever as they are great for snacks.

Are you dining out? Hit the salad bar. There are so many delicious salads you can try, especially when you're in a good restaurant. This is actually a great alternative if you don't feel like making your own salads.

You can place them on your kitchen counter. Got some in the fridge? Set it up, so they're right in front of you when you open it. Why? When you can see your fruits and veggies, you're more likely to eat them.

Be sure to stock up on all sorts of fresh, frozen, and canned fruits and vegetables so you can enjoy them weekly. Remember your veggies make up most of your meals, so the last thing you want to do is run out.

How do I tell which fruit and veggies are good and fresh? And how do I store them?

Easy. Look for veggies and fruit which aren't shriveled, don't look bruised, don't have mold and don't seem slimy. The smell is a good way to tell if something isn't fresh. If it smells off, don't buy it. The produce workers in the store can also help you decide which items to go for. You could request information on storing the fruit and veggies that you choose.

When it comes to most fruits and veggies, you can't really buy large amounts of them. If you're not using all of it within the next few days or at least within the week, they're likely to go bad. So make sure you only buy enough to last you a few days. If you want fruits and veggies which will keep longer, then stock up on the frozen kind.

When you're shopping, make sure you keep the fruits and veggies on top of everything else in your cart. If you put heavy stuff on it, some of the fruit will bruise and the vegetables may get damaged as well.

At home, keep as much of your produce in the crisper compartment of your fridge as you can as they will keep longer. Got some already cut veggies and fruit? Keep them in the fridge.

Rather than wash your veggies and fruit before putting them away, opt to wash them right before you eat or use them instead. This will help them stay as fresh as they can for as long as possible.

If you've got some unripe fruit, put them in a brown paper bag (make sure it's only closed loosely). Better yet, get a ripening bowl.

Everyone says carbs make you gain weight. Why are they part of the DASH Diet?

Not all carbs are created equal. Carbs are not all that bad when taken in moderation. It is very natural to be concerned about your carb intake if you are trying to lose weight. When you think of carbs, you probably think of bread, white rice, and pasta. Guess what?

Fruits are carbs. Veggies are carbs too.

So what is the difference? If your end goal is to lose weight and eat right then, you'll find carbs which have fiber and lots of other great nutrients are good for you. I'm talking about whole grains, veggies, and fruit. They're packed with phytochemicals, minerals and lots of vitamins. These carbs are complex carbs. Yes, they still break down into sugar like the simple carbs, but because of their complexity, they do so slowly. As a result, your blood sugar levels won't spike hard and fast like when you eat plain sugar, making it safe to have these carbs.

It's hard to do the DASH Diet when I'm on the road. Any advice?

Yes, it's going to be a bit more challenging when you're on the move to focus on your DASH meal plan. You're going to have to try. First things first -

control your portions, so you're not eating too much. Find menu items that work with the DASH Diet. If you can't find options, then really control your portions as best as you can.

Also, it's more important than ever that you stick with your exercise routine. You need to be active as often as you can. Take time to explore where you are on foot. Take the stairs when you can. Go hiking. Hit the gym if you're staying in a hotel. Do whatever you can to move your body!

How to follow DASH when eating out?

When eating out at restaurants, these tips can help you order the best options.

Try foods like:

- Grilled, roasted, broiled menu items
- Fresh fruits and vegetables as sides
- Spices and fresh herbs, which do not contain sodium (basil, garlic, curry powder, etc.)
- Fresh vegetables for pizza and burger toppings
- Vegetarian dishes
- Fresh fruits or sorbets for dessert

Limit or avoid foods that tend to be higher in sodium:

- Meats that are fried, smoked, cured, or processed
- Condiments like mustard, ketchup, pickles, and soy sauce
- Most soups
- Additives like MSG
- Dishes like rice pilaf, casserole-style dishes, charcuterie plates (cheese, cured meats, olives)

Don't be afraid to:

- Ask for the nutrition information (specifically sodium) for any foods you are unsure about.
- Ask that less or no salt be added to your dish.
- Ask for dressings and sauces on the side to help control the amount of sodium you'll be ingesting.
- Most importantly… taste your food before you season it!
- Don't let high blood pressure stop you from enjoying dining out with friend and family. With these easy changes, you can manage your health deliciously! Work with your doctor and/or a registered dietitian to stay on track with a diet to lower blood pressure.

Chapter 8. DASH DIET RECIPES

Here are over 80 delicious and easy to prepare recipes for your enjoyment. They are broken down into recipes of Breakfast & Smoothies, Appetizers, Vegetarian & Vegan Mains, Poultry & Seafood Mains, Beef & Pork Mains, Snacks, Sides & Desserts, Legumes & Grains.

Enjoy.

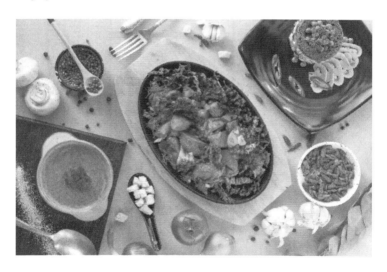

Picture source: unsplash.com

BREAKFASTS & SMOOTHIES

Microwave Quiche in a Mug

Preparation Time: 2 minutes
Cook Time: 3 minutes
Servings: 1

Ingredients

- ½ cup chopped frozen spinach, thawed and drained (or ½ cup packed fresh spinach)
- 1 large egg
- ⅓ cup low-fat milk
- 1 teaspoon olive oil
- Freshly ground black pepper
- ½ slice whole-grain bread, torn into small pieces

Directions

1. If using fresh spinach, place it in a mug with 2 tablespoons of water. Cover with a paper towel and microwave for 1 minute. Remove from microwave and drain the water from the spinach before adding it back to the mug. If using frozen spinach, make sure it is completely thawed and drained.
2. Crack the egg into the mug with the spinach and add the milk, olive oil, and pepper. Whisk until thoroughly mixed.
3. Add bread and stir in gently, but do not whisk.

4. Place the mug in the microwave and cook on high for 1 minute until the egg is cooked, and quiche is slightly puffed.
5. Serve immediately.

Nutritional Values: Per Serving Total Calories: 216; Total Fat: 11g; Saturated Fat: 3g; Cholesterol: 191mg; Sodium: 268mg; Potassium: 352mg; Total Carbohydrates: 18g; Fiber: 4g; Sugars: 5g; Protein: 14g

Avocado And Egg Toast

Preparation Time: 5 Minutes
Cook Time: 5 Minutes
Servings: 1

Ingredients

- 2 eggs
- 2 slices whole-grain bread
- 1 small avocado
- 1 teaspoon freshly squeezed lime juice
- Freshly ground black pepper

Directions

1. Toast bread and cook the eggs to personal preference.
2. Peel and mash avocado with the lime juice and pepper.
3. Spread avocado evenly on each slice of toast, then top each with a fried egg.
4. Serve immediately.

Nutritional Values: Per Serving Total Calories: 612; Total Fat: 38g; Saturated Fat: 7g; Cholesterol: 372mg; Sodium: 535mg; Potassium: 1,015mg; Total Carbohydrates: 50g; Fiber: 18g; Sugars: 7g; Protein: 24g

Steel-Cut Oats with Blueberries and Almonds

Preparation Time: 10 Minutes
Cook Time: 17 Minutes
Servings: 4

Ingredients

- 1 cup nonfat or low-fat milk
- 1 cup of water
- 1 teaspoon ground cinnamon
- 1 cup steel-cut oats
- 1 cup blueberries
- ½ cup sliced almonds

Directions

1. In a medium saucepan over medium heat, whisk together milk, water, and cinnamon.
2. When the mixture starts to come to a boil, add steel-cut oats and bring to a boil.
3. Reduce heat to low and simmer for 15 minutes.
4. About 2 minutes before the end of cooking time, add in blueberries and almonds and stir well.
5. Serve immediately.

Nutritional Values: Per Serving Total Calories: 268; Total Fat: 10g; Saturated Fat: 1g; Cholesterol: 1mg; Sodium: 28mg; Potassium: 241mg; Total Carbohydrates: 39g; Fiber: 7g; Sugars: 7g; Protein: 11g

Peaches and Greens Smoothie

Preparation Time: 5 minutes
Servings: 1

Ingredients

- 2 cups fresh spinach (or ⅓ cup frozen)
- 1 cup frozen peaches (or fresh, pitted)
- 1 cup ice
- ½ cup nonfat or low-fat milk
- ½ cup plain nonfat or low-fat Greek yogurt
- ½ teaspoon vanilla extract
- Optional: calorie-free sweetener of choice

Directions

1. Add all of the ingredients to a blender and process until smooth.
2. Enjoy immediately.

Nutritional Values: Per Serving Total Calories: 191; Total Fat: 0g; Saturated Fat: 0g; Cholesterol: 7mg; Sodium: 157mg; Potassium: 984mg; Total Carbohydrates: 30g; Fiber: 3g; Sugars: 23g; Protein: 18g

Strawberry Yogurt Smoothie

Preparation Time: 5 minutes
Servings: 1

Ingredients

- 1 cup plain nonfat or low-fat Greek yogurt
- 1 cup frozen strawberries
- 1 cup ice
- ½ cup nonfat or low-fat milk
- ½ orange, peeled
- ½ frozen banana

Directions

1. Add all of the ingredients to a blender and process until smooth.
2. Enjoy immediately.

Nutritional Values: Per Serving Total Calories: 305; Total Fat: 1g; Saturated Fat: 0g; Cholesterol: 13mg; Sodium: 170mg; Potassium: 1,284mg; Total Carbohydrates: 52g; Fiber: 6g; Sugars: 37g; Protein: 29g

Peanut Butter and Banana Smoothie

Preparation Time: 5 Minutes
Servings:1

Ingredients

- 1 cup nonfat or low-fat milk
- 1 cup ice
- ¼ cup plain nonfat or low-fat Greek yogurt
- 1 frozen banana, sliced
- 1 tablespoon peanut butter

Directions

1. Add all of the ingredients to a blender and process until smooth.
2. Enjoy immediately.

Nutritional Values: Per Serving Total Calories: 313; Total Fat: 9g; Saturated Fat: 2g; Cholesterol: 8mg; Sodium: 136mg; Potassium: 1,037mg; Total Carbohydrates: 45g; Fiber: 5g; Sugars: 30g; Protein: 19g

Blueberry-Oatmeal Muffin in a Mug

Preparation Time: 1 Minute
Cook Time: 1 Minute
Servings: 1

Ingredients

- ½ cup rolled oats
- 1 egg
- 2 tablespoons nonfat or low-fat milk
- ⅓ cup blueberries
- Cooking spray
- *Optional:* calorie-free sweetener of choice

Directions

1. Spray a large mug or small ramekin with cooking spray.
2. Add the oats, egg, and milk, and stir to combine. Gently fold in the blueberries.
3. Place in the microwave and cook on high for 1 minute, being careful to watch as it could overflow. If the muffin does not look firm, place back in for 30 seconds at a time.
4. Once ready, flip mug upside down onto a plate, slice, and enjoy.

Nutritional Values: Per Serving Total Calories: 259; Total Fat: 8g; Saturated Fat: 2g; Cholesterol: 187mg; Sodium: 87mg; Potassium: 159mg; Total Carbohydrates: 36g; Fiber: 5g; Sugars: 8g; Protein: 13g

Cantaloupe Smoothie

Preparation Time: 5 Minutes
Servings: 2

Ingredients

- ½ cup nonfat or low-fat milk
- 1 frozen banana, sliced
- 1 (5.3-ounce) carton vanilla fat-free Greek yogurt
- ½ cup ice
- 1 teaspoon honey
- 2½ cups (1-inch) cubed and peeled frozen cantaloupe

Directions

1. In a food processor or blender, blend the first 5 ingredients until the consistency is smooth.
2. Add frozen cantaloupe pieces to the mixture in the blender and process until the desired consistency is reached.
3. Enjoy

Nutritional Values: Per Serving Total Calories: 214; Total Fat: 1g; Saturated Fat: 0g; Cholesterol: 4mg; Sodium: 67mg; Potassium: 994mg; Total Carbohydrates: 46g; Fiber: 3g; Sugars: 38g; Protein: 11g

Cranberry Orange Muffins

Preparation Time: 10 minutes
Cooking Time: 20 minutes
Servings: 4

Ingredients:

- 8 ounces fat-free plain Greek yogurt
- 2 eggs
- 1/4 cup canola oil
- 1/2 cup granulated sugar
- 1/4 cup brown sugar
- 2 tablespoons unsweetened orange juice concentrate
- 2 tablespoons orange zest
- 2 teaspoons vanilla
- 1 3/4 cup all-purpose flour
- 1/4 cup flaxseed meal
- 1 teaspoon baking powder
- 1 teaspoon baking soda
- 1/8 teaspoon salt
- 1/2 teaspoon cinnamon
- 1 1/2 cups fresh or frozen cranberries

Directions

1. Grease a muffin tin with cooking spray. Set the oven to 350°F.

2. Whisk eggs with sugars, oil, yogurt, orange zest, vanilla, and orange juice in a bowl.

3. Combine flaxseed with baking powder, cinnamon, salt, flour, and baking soda in another bowl.

4. Mix the dry and wet mixtures together in the mixing bowl at low speed until well mixed.

5. Fold in cranberries after 2 minutes of mixing.

6. Scoop the batter into muffin cups.

7. Bake for 20 minutes until golden brown.

8. Serve with desired garnish.

Nutritional Values: Per Serving Total Calories: 210; Total Fat: 24.7g; Saturated Fat: 8g; Cholesterol: 0mg; Sodium: 840 mg; Potassium: 994mg; Total Carbohydrates: 60g; Fiber: 6g; Sugars: 41.1 g; Protein: 13.5g

Raspberry Chocolate Scones

Preparation Time: 7 minutes
Cooking Time: 12 minutes
Servings: 4

Ingredients:

* 1 cup whole-wheat pastry flour
* 1 cup all-purpose flour
* 1 tablespoon baking powder
* 1/4 teaspoon baking soda
* 1/3 cup trans-fat-free buttery spread
* 1/2 cup fresh or frozen raspberries
* 1/4 cup miniature chocolate chips
* 1 cup plus 2 tablespoons plain fat-free yogurt
* 2 tablespoons honey
* 1/2 teaspoon sugar
* 1/4 teaspoon cinnamon

Directions

1. Preheat the oven to 400°F.
2. Combine flours with baking soda and baking powder in a mixing bowl.
3. Cut the butter into the dry mixture. Blend until it forms a crumbly mixture.
4. Fold in chocolate chips and berries.
5. Pour in honey and yogurt and stir the mixture gently to form a crumbly batter.

6. Knead the dough on a flowered surface and then spread it into ½ inch thick circle.

7. Slice the sheet into 12 wedges. Arrange them on a greased baking sheet.

8. Sprinkle the sugar and cinnamon mixture on top.

9. Bake them for 12 minutes at 400 degrees F.

10. Serve and enjoy.

Nutritional Values: Calories 149; Total Fat 13.7 g; Saturated Fat 12.7 g; Cholesterol 78 mg; Sodium 141 mg; Total Carbohydrates 22.9 g; Fiber 3.2 g; Sugar 1.3 g; Protein 4.2 g.

Whole-Wheat Pretzels

Preparation Time: 10 minutes
Cook Time: 15 minutes
Servings: 4

Ingredients:

- 1 package active dry yeast
- 2 teaspoons brown sugar
- 1/2 teaspoon kosher salt
- 1 1/2 cups warm water
- 1 cup bread flour
- 3 cups whole-wheat flour
- 1 tablespoon olive oil
- 1/2 cup wheat gluten
- Cooking spray, as needed
- 1/4 cup baking soda
- 1 egg white or 1/4 cup egg substitute
- 1 tablespoon of sesame, poppy, or sunflower seeds

Directions

1. Preheat the oven to 450°F.
2. Mix yeast with salt, sugar, and water in a bowl and let it rest for 5 minutes.
3. Combine flours with gluten and olive oil in a processor.

4. Mix in the yeast mixture and knead the dough until smooth.

5. Cover the dough in the bowl with a plastic sheet and keep it in a warm place for 1 hour until the dough is raised.

6. Punch down the dough and then divide the dough into 14 pieces.

7. Roll each piece into long ropes and make a pretzel shape out of the dough rope.

8. Boil 10 cups water with ¼ cup baking soda in a pot. Place the pretzels in the water.

9. Cook each pretzel for 30 seconds then immediately transfer them to a baking pan lined with parchment paper using a slotted spoon.

10. Brush each pretzel with whisked egg whites and drizzle sesame, sunflower, and poppy seeds on top.

11. Bake for 15 minutes at 450 degrees F

12. Serve.

Nutritional Values: Calories 148; Total Fat 12.8 g; Saturated Fat 10.6 g; Cholesterol 112 mg; Sodium 32 mg; Total Carbohydrates 31.5 g; Fiber 4.2 g; Sugar 2.5 g; Protein 7.6 g

APPETIZER RECIPES

Smoked Trout Spread

Preparation Time: 5 minutes
Cook Time: 0 minutes
Servings: 4

Ingredients:

- 1/4-pound smoked trout fillet or other white fish
- 1/2 cup fat-free cottage cheese
- 1/4 cup red onion, diced
- 2 teaspoons freshly squeezed lemon juice
- 1 teaspoon hot pepper sauce
- 1/2 teaspoon Worcestershire sauce
- 1 celery stalk, chopped

Directions

1. Remove skin on trout fillet and using a fork break into small pieces.
2. Blend trout with cottage cheese, lemon juice, Worcestershire sauce, red onion, and hot pepper sauce in a food processor.
3. Continue blending until smooth.
4. Fold in diced celery. Cover the spread.
5. Refrigerate and serve.

Nutritional Values: Calories 201; Total Fat 24.5 g; Saturated Fat 3.7 g; Cholesterol 151 mg Sodium 514 mg Total Carbohydrates 9.3 g Fiber 1.3 g Sugar 0 g Protein 3.9 g

Apples with Dip

Preparation Time: 5 minutes
Cooking Time: 0 minutes
Servings: 4

Ingredients:

- 8 ounces low-free cream cheese
- 2 tablespoons brown sugar
- 1 1/2 teaspoons vanilla extract
- 2 tablespoons peanuts, coarsely chopped
- 4 medium or 8 small apples, cored and sliced
- 1/2 cup orange juice

Directions

1. Soften the cream cheese for 5 minutes at room temperature.
2. Combine vanilla with cream cheese and brown sugar in a bowl until smooth.
3. Fold in peanuts.
4. Serve this dip with sliced apples. If desired, garnish with a drizzle of orange juice on top.

Nutritional Values: Calories 110; Total Fat 9.8 g; Saturated Fat 1.4 g; Cholesterol 20 mg; Sodium 119 mg; Total Carbohydrates 11.3 g; Fiber 0.5 g; Sugar 1.2 g; Protein 7.6 g.

Spicy Roasted Broccoli

Preparation Time: 10 minutes
Cooking Time: 25 minutes
Servings: 4

Ingredients:

- 1 1/4 pounds broccoli, chopped (about 8 cups)
- 4 tablespoons olive oil
- 1/2 teaspoon salt-free seasoning blend
- 1/4 teaspoon freshly ground black pepper
- 4 cloves garlic, peeled and minced

Directions

1. Preheat oven to 450°F.
2. Toss broccoli with 2 tablespoons olive oil in a bowl.
3. Mix pepper with the seasoning blend. Spread broccoli evenly on a baking sheet and sprinkle with the seasoning mixture.
4. Bake for 15 minutes.
5. In a small bowl, blend the remainder of the olive oil with garlic.
6. Top the baked broccoli with the garlic mixture and toss well.
7. Bake the broccoli again for 10 minutes.
8. Serve.

Nutritional Values: Calories 183; Total Fat 16.3 g; Saturated Fat 3.5 g; Cholesterol 142 mg; Sodium 144 mg; Total Carbohydrates 2.3g; Fiber 1.3 g; Sugar 1.7 g; Protein 12.3 g

VEGETARIAN & VEGAN MAINS

Black-Bean and Vegetable Burrito

Preparation Time: 10 minutes
Cook Time: 15 minutes
Servings: 4

Ingredients

- ½ tablespoon olive oil
- 2 red or green bell peppers, cored and chopped
- 1 zucchini or summer squash, diced
- ½ teaspoon chili powder
- 1 teaspoon cumin
- Freshly ground black pepper
- 2 (15-ounce) cans black beans, drained and rinsed
- 1 cup cherry tomatoes, halved
- 4 (8-inch) whole-wheat tortillas
- *Optional for serving:* spinach, sliced avocado, chopped scallions or hot sauce

Directions

1. Heat the oil in a large sauté pan over medium heat. Add the bell peppers and sauté until crisp-tender (about 4 minutes).

2. Add the zucchini, chili powder, cumin, and black pepper to taste and continue to sauté until the vegetables are tender (about 5 minutes).

3. Add the black beans and cherry tomatoes. Cook Time: until the tomatoes soften, the beans are heated through, and most of the moisture has evaporated (about 5 minutes).

4. Divide between 4 burritos and serve topped with optional ingredients as desired.

5. Enjoy immediately.

Nutritional Values: Per Serving Total Calories: 311; Total Fat: 6g; Saturated Fat: 1g; Cholesterol: 0mg; Sodium: 499mg; Potassium: 400mg; Total Carbohydrates: 52g; Fiber: 21g; Sugars: 1g; Protein: 19g

Baked Eggs In Avocado

Preparation Time: 10 minutes
Cook Time: 15 minutes
Servings: 4

Ingredients

- 2 avocados
- Juice of 2 limes
- Freshly ground black pepper
- 4 eggs
- 2 (8-inch) whole-wheat or corn tortillas, warmed
- *Optional for serving:* halved cherry tomatoes and chopped cilantro

Directions

1. Adjust oven rack to the middle position and preheat the oven to 450°F.
2. Cut each avocado in half and remove the pit. Using a spoon, scrape out the center of each halved avocado so that it is large enough to accommodate an egg (about 1½ tablespoons). Squeeze lime juice over the avocados and season with black pepper to taste. Place on a baking sheet. Break an egg into the center of each avocado. Don't worry if some of the white spills out, as long as the yolk is intact.

3. Bake until whites are set and the yolk is runny (10 to 15 minutes).

4. Remove from oven and garnish with optional cilantro and cherry tomatoes and serve with warm tortillas.

Nutritional Values: Per Serving Total Calories: 534; Total Fat: 39g; Saturated Fat: 8g; Cholesterol: 372mg; Sodium: 462mg; Potassium: 1,095mg; Total Carbohydrates: 30g; Fiber: 20g; Sugars: 3g; Protein: 23g

Black-Bean Soup

Preparation Time: 5 minutes
Cook Time: 20 minutes
Servings: 4

Directions

- 1 yellow onion
- 1 tablespoon olive oil
- 2 (15-ounce) cans black beans, drained and rinsed
- 1 cup diced fresh tomatoes
- 5 cups low-sodium vegetable broth
- ¼ teaspoon freshly ground black pepper
- ¼ cup chopped fresh cilantro

Directions

1. In a large saucepan, cook the onion in the olive oil over medium heat until softened (about 4 to 5 minute)s.
2. Add the black beans, tomatoes, vegetable broth, and black pepper. Bring to a boil. Reduce heat and simmer for about 15 minutes.
3. Remove from the heat and working in batches ladle the soup into a blender and process until somewhat smooth. Return the soup to the pot, add the cilantro and heat until warmed through.
4. Serve immediately.

Nutritional Values: Per Serving Total Calories: 234; Total Fat: 5g; Saturated Fat: 1g; Cholesterol: 0mg; Sodium: 363mg; Potassium: 145mg; Total Carbohydrates: 37g; Fiber: 13g; Sugars: 3g; Protein: 11g

Loaded Baked Sweet Potatoes

Preparation Time: 10 minutes
Cook Time: 20 minutes
Servings: 4

Ingredients

- 4 sweet potatoes
- ½ cup nonfat or low-fat plain Greek yogurt
- Freshly ground black pepper
- 1 teaspoon olive oil
- 1 red bell pepper, cored and diced
- ½ red onion, diced
- 1 teaspoon ground cumin
- 1 (15-ounce) can chickpeas, drained and rinsed

Directions

1. Poke holes in the potatoes with a fork.
Cook on your microwave's potato setting until potatoes are soft and cooked through (about 8 to 10 minutes for 4 potatoes).
2. Combine the yogurt and black pepper in a small bowl and mix well.
3. Heat the oil in a medium pot over medium heat. Add bell pepper, onion, cumin, and additional black pepper to taste.
4. Add the chickpeas, stir to combine, and heat through (about 5 minutes).

5. Slice the potatoes lengthwise down the middle and top each half with a portion of the bean mixture followed by 1 to 2 tablespoons of the yogurt.

6. Serve immediately.

Nutritional Values: Per Serving Total Calories: 264; Total Fat: 2g; Saturated Fat: 0g; Cholesterol: 1mg; Sodium: 124mg; Potassium: 428mg; Total Carbohydrates: 51g; Fiber: 10g; Sugars: 1g; Protein: 11g

White Beans with Spinach and Pan-Roasted Tomatoes

Preparation Time: 15 minutes
Cook Time: 10 minutes
Servings: 2

Ingredients

- 1 tablespoon olive oil
- 4 small plum tomatoes, halved lengthwise
- 10 ounces frozen spinach, defrosted and squeezed of excess water
- 2 garlic cloves, thinly sliced
- 2 tablespoons water
- ¼ teaspoon freshly ground black pepper
- 1 (15-ounce) can white beans, drained and rinsed
- Juice of 1 lemon

Directions

1. Heat the oil in a large skillet over medium high heat. Add the tomatoes, cut-side down. Cook Time: shaking the pan occasionally, until browned and starting to soften (about 3 to 5 minutes). Turn and cook for 1 minute more. Transfer to a plate.
2. Reduce heat to medium and add the spinach, garlic, water, and pepper to the skillet.

Toss while cooking until the spinach is heated through (2 to 3 minutes).
3. Return the tomatoes to the skillet. Add the white beans and lemon juice, and toss until heated through (about 1 to 2 minutes).

Nutritional Values: Per Serving Total Calories: 293; Total Fat: 9g; Saturated Fat: 1g; Cholesterol: 0mg; Sodium: 267mg; Potassium: 648mg; Total Carbohydrates: 43g; Fiber: 16g; Sugars: 1g; Protein: 15g

Black-Eyed Peas and Greens Power Salad

Preparation Time: 5 minutes
Cook Time: 6 minutes
Servings: 2

Ingredients

- 1 tablespoon olive oil
- 3 cups purple cabbage, chopped
- 5 cups baby spinach
- 1 cup shredded carrots
- 1 (15-ounce) can black-eyed peas, drained and rinsed
- Juice of ½ lemon
- Salt
- Freshly ground black pepper

Directions

1. In a medium pan, add the oil and cabbage and sauté for 1 to 2 minutes on medium heat.
2. Add in your spinach. Cover and cook for 3 to 4 minutes on medium heat until greens are wilted.
3. Remove from the heat and add to a large bowl.
4. Add in the carrots, black-eyed peas, and a splash of lemon juice.
5. Season with salt and pepper, if desired.
6. Toss together and serve.

Nutritional Values: Per Serving Total Calories: 320; Total Fat: 9g; Saturated Fat: 1g; Cholesterol: 0mg; Sodium: 351mg; Potassium: 544mg; Total Carbohydrates: 49g; Fiber: 18g; Sugars: 10g; Protein: 16g

Butternut-Squash Macaroni and Cheese

Preparation Time: 10 minutes
Cook Time: 20 minutes
Servings: 2

Ingredients

- 1 cup whole-wheat ziti macaroni
- 2 cups peeled and cubed butternut squash
- 1 cup nonfat or low-fat milk, divided
- Freshly ground black pepper
- 1 teaspoon Dijon mustard
- 1 tablespoon olive oil
- ¼ cup shredded low-fat cheddar cheese

Directions

1. Cook the pasta al dente.
2. In a medium saucepan, add the butternut squash and ½ cup milk and place cook at medium-high. Season with black pepper. Bring to a simmer. Reduce heat to low and cover. Cook until fork tender (8 to 10 minutes).
3. In a blender, add squash and Dijon mustard. Purée until smooth.
4. Place a large sauté pan over medium heat and add olive oil. Add the squash purée and remaining ½ cup of milk. Bring to a simmer.

Cook until thickened (about 5 minutes). Add the cheese and stir to combine.

5. Add the pasta to the sauté pan and stir to combine.

6. Serve immediately.

Nutritional Values: Per Serving Total Calories: 373; Total Fat: 10g; Saturated Fat: 2g; Cholesterol: 8mg; Sodium: 193mg; Potassium: 783mg; Total Carbohydrates: 59g; Fiber: 10g; Sugars: 8g; Protein: 14g

Pasta with Tomatoes and Peas

Preparation Time: 10 minutes
Cook Time: 15 minutes
Servings: 2

Ingredients

- ½ cup whole-grain pasta of choice
- 8 cups water, plus ¼ for finishing
- 1 cup frozen peas
- 1 tablespoon olive oil
- 1 cup cherry tomatoes, halved
- ¼ teaspoon freshly ground black pepper
- 1 teaspoon dried basil
- ¼ cup grated Parmesan cheese (low-sodium)

Directions

1. Cook the pasta al dente.
2. Add the water to the same pot you used to cook the pasta. Bring the water to a boil and add the peas. Cook until tender, but still firm (about 5 minutes). Drain and set aside.
3. Heat the oil in a large skillet over medium heat. Add the cherry tomatoes. Put a lid on the skillet and let the tomatoes soften for about 5 minutes, stirring a few times.
4. Season with black pepper and basil.

5. Toss in the pasta, peas, and ¼ cup of water. Stir and remove from the heat.

6. Serve topped with Parmesan cheese.

Nutritional Values: Per Serving Total Calories: 266; Total Fat: 12g; Saturated Fat: 4g; Cholesterol: 10mg; Sodium: 320mg; Potassium: 313mg; Total Carbohydrates: 30g; Fiber: 6g; Sugars: 5g; Protein: 13g

Healthy Vegetable Fried Rice

Preparation Time: 5 minutes
Cook Time: 10 minutes
Servings: 4

Ingredients

For The Sauce:
- ⅓ cup garlic vinegar
- 1½ tablespoons dark molasses
- 1 teaspoon onion powder

For The Fried Rice:
- 1 teaspoon olive oil
- 2 whole eggs plus 4 egg whites, lightly beaten
- 1 cup frozen mixed vegetables
- 1 cup frozen edamame
- 2 cups cooked brown rice

Directions

To make the sauce
Prepare the sauce by combining the garlic vinegar, molasses, and onion powder in a glass jar. Shake well.

To make the fried rice
1. Heat oil in a large wok or skillet over medium-high heat. Add eggs and egg whites and let cook until the eggs are set (about 1 minute). Break eggs

into small pieces with a spatula or. Add frozen mixed vegetables and frozen edamame. Cook for 4 minutes, stirring frequently.

2. Add the brown rice and sauce to the vegetable-and-egg mixture. Cook for 5 minutes or until heated through.

3. Serve immediately.

Nutritional Values: Per Serving Total Calories: 210; Total Fat: 6g; Saturated Fat: 1g; Cholesterol: 93mg; Sodium: 113mg; Potassium: 183mg; Total Carbohydrates: 28g; Fiber: 3g; Sugars: 6g; Protein: 13g

Portobello-Mushroom Cheeseburgers

Preparation Time: 5 minutes
Cook Time: 10 minutes
Servings: 4

Ingredients

- 4 Portobello mushrooms, caps removed and brushed clean
- 1 tablespoon olive oil
- ½ teaspoon freshly ground black pepper
- 1 tablespoon red wine vinegar
- 4 slices reduced-fat Swiss cheese, sliced thin
- 4 whole-wheat 100-calorie sandwich thins
- ½ avocado, sliced thin

Directions

1. Heat a skillet or grill pan over medium-high heat. Clean the mushrooms and remove the stems. Brush each cap with olive oil and sprinkle with black pepper. Place in skillet, cap-side up and cook for about 4 minutes. Flip and cook for another 4 minutes.
2. Sprinkle with the red wine vinegar and turn over. Add the cheese and cook for 2 more minutes. For optimal melting, place a lid loosely over the pan.

3. Toast the sandwich thins. Create your burgers by topping each with sliced avocado.
4. Enjoy immediately.

Nutritional Values: Per Serving Total Calories: 245; Total Fat: 12g; Saturated Fat: 3g; Cholesterol: 15mg; Sodium: 266mg; Potassium: 507mg; Total Carbohydrates: 28g; Fiber: 8g; Sugars: 4g; Protein: 14g

Baked Chickpea-and-Rosemary Omelet

Preparation Time: 10 minutes
Cook Time: 15 minutes
Servings: 2

Ingredients

- ½ tablespoon olive oil
- 4 eggs
- ¼ cup grated Parmesan cheese
- 1 (15-ounce) can chickpeas, drained and rinsed
- 2 cups packed baby spinach
- 1 cup button mushrooms, chopped
- 2 sprigs rosemary, leaves picked (or 2 teaspoons dried rosemary)
- Salt
- Freshly ground black pepper

Directions

1. Preheat the oven to 400°F and place a baking tray on the middle shelf.
2. Line an 8-inch springform pan with baking paper and grease generously with olive oil. If you don't have a springform pan, grease an oven-safe skillet (or cast-iron skillet) with olive oil.
3. Lightly whisk together the eggs and Parmesan.
4. Place chickpeas in the pan. Layer the spinach and mushrooms on top of the beans. Pour the egg

mixture on top and scatter the rosemary. Season to taste with salt and pepper.

5. Place the pan on the preheated tray and bake until golden and puffy and the center feels firm and springy (about 15 minutes).

6. Remove from the oven, slice, and serve immediately.

Nutritional Values: Per Serving Total Calories: 418; Total Fat: 19g; Saturated Fat: 6g; Cholesterol: 382mg; Sodium: 595mg; Potassium: 273mg; Total Carbohydrates: 33g; Fiber: 12g; Sugars: 2g; Protein: 30g

Easy Chickpea Veggie Burgers

Preparation Time:: 10 minutes
Cook Time: 20 minutes
Servings: 4

Ingredients

- 1 15-ounce can chickpeas, drained and rinsed
- ½ cup frozen spinach, thawed
- ⅓ cup rolled oats
- 1 teaspoon garlic powder
- 1 teaspoon onion powder

Directions

1. Preheat oven to 400°F. Grease a sheet or line one with parchment paper and set aside.
2. In a mixing bowl, add half of the beans and mash with a fork until fairly smooth. Set aside.
3. Add the remaining half of the beans, spinach, oats, and spices to a food processor or blender and blend until puréed. Add the mixture to the bowl of mashed beans and stir until well combined.
4. Divide mixture into 4 equal portions and shape into patties. Bake for 7 to 10 minutes. Carefully turn over and bake for another 7 to 10 minutes or until crusty on the outside.
5. Place on a whole grain bun with your favorite toppings.

Nutritional Values: Per Serving Total Calories: 118; Total Fat: 1g; Saturated Fat: 0g; Cholesterol: 7mg; Sodium: 108mg; Potassium: 83mg; Total Carbohydrates: 21g; Fiber: 7g; Sugars: 0g; Protein: 7g

Rotelle Pasta with Sun-Dried Tomato

Preparation Time: 10 minutes
Cooking Time: 20 minutes
Servings: 4

Ingredients

- 2 tablespoons olive oil
- 4 garlic cloves, mashed
- 1/3 cup dry-packed sun-dried tomatoes, soaked in water to rehydrate, drained and chopped
- 1 3/4 cups unsalted vegetable broth
- 8 ounces uncooked whole-wheat rotelle pasta
- 1/2 cup sliced black olives (about 15 medium olives)
- 1/2 cup chopped fresh parsley
- 4 teaspoons parmesan cheese

Directions

1. Preheat olive oil in a skillet over medium heat.
2. Sauté garlic for 30 seconds. Then add tomatoes and broth.
3. Cover the mixture and then simmer for 10 minutes.
4. Fill a pot with water and boil pasta in it for 10 minutes until al dente.
5. Drain the pasta and keep it aside.

6. Add parsley and olives to the tomato mixture and mix well.

7. Serve the plate with tomato sauce and add 1 teaspoon parmesan cheese on top.

Nutritional Values: Calories 335 Total Fat 4.4 g; Saturated Fat 2.1 g; Cholesterol 10 mg; Sodium 350 mg; Total Carbohydrates 31.2 g; Fiber 2.7 g; Sugar 0.6 g; Protein 7.3 g

Rice Noodles with Spring Vegetables

Preparation Time: 5 minutes
Cooking Time: 10 minutes
Servings: 2

Ingredients

- 1 package (8 ounces) rice noodles
- 1 tablespoon peanut oil
- 1 tablespoon sesame oil
- 1 tablespoon grated fresh ginger
- 2 garlic cloves, finely chopped
- 2 tablespoons low-sodium soy sauce
- 1 cup small broccoli florets
- 1 cup fresh bean sprouts
- 8 cherry tomatoes, halved
- 1 cup chopped fresh spinach
- 2 scallions, chopped
- Crushed red chili flakes (optional)

Directions

1. Boil the noodles in a pot filled with water for 6 minutes until al dente and then drain it thoroughly.
2. Preheat oil in a wok and sauté garlic and ginger for 30 secs.
3. Stir in remaining ingredients, including vegetables and noodles.

4. Toss the mixture well and then serve with crushed chili flakes on top.

Nutritional Values: Calories 205; Total Fat 1.1 g; Saturated Fat 2.8 g; Cholesterol 110 mg; Sodium 749 mg; Total Carbohydrates 12.9 g; Fiber 0.2 g; Sugar 0.2 g; Protein 63.5 g.

Pasta with Pumpkin Sauce

Preparation Time: 5 minutes
Cooking Time: 20 minutes
Servings: 4

Ingredients

- 2 cups whole-wheat bow tie pasta
- 2 teaspoons olive oil
- 1 medium onion, chopped
- 4 cloves garlic, minced
- 8 ounces fresh mushrooms, sliced
- 1 cup low-sodium chicken or vegetable broth
- 1 can (15 ounces) pumpkin
- 1/2 teaspoon rubbed sage
- 1/8 teaspoon salt
- 1/4 teaspoon ground black pepper
- 1/4 cup grated Parmesan cheese
- 1 tablespoon dried parsley flakes

Directions

1. Boil the pasta per the given instructions on the box and drain it.
2. Preheat olive oil in a skillet and sauté onions, garlic, and mushrooms for 10 minutes.
3. Stir in pumpkin, salt, pepper, broth, and sage.
4. Cook the mixture on medium heat for 8 minutes.

5. Add cooked pasta to the pumpkin sauce.
6. Garnish with Parmesan cheese and parsley.
7. Serve.

Nutritional Values: Calories 197; Total Fat 3.5 g;
Saturated Fat 0.5 g; Cholesterol 162 mg; Sodium
142 mg; Total Carbohydrates 3.6g; Fiber 0.4 g;
Sugar 0.5 g; Protein 21.5 g

Fresh Puttanesca with Brown Rice

Preparation Time: 10 minutes
Cooking Time: 0 minutes
Servings: 4

Ingredients:

- 4 cups chopped ripe plum tomatoes
- 4 Kalamata olives, pitted and sliced
- 4 green olives, pitted and sliced
- 1 1/2 tablespoons capers, rinsed and drained
- 1 tablespoon minced garlic
- 1 tablespoon olive oil
- 1/4 cup chopped fresh basil
- 1 tablespoon minced fresh parsley
- 1/8 teaspoon red pepper flakes
- 3 cups cooked brown rice

Directions

1. Mix tomatoes with capers, garlic, oil, olives, parsley, red pepper flakes, and basil in a bowl.
2. Let this mixture refrigerate for 20 minutes.
3. Serve over boiled brown rice.

Nutritional Values: Calories 250; Total Fat 7.5 g; Saturated Fat 1.1 g; Cholesterol 20 mg Sodium 97 mg; Total Carbohydrates 21.4 g; Fiber 0 g; Sugar 0 g; Protein 5.1g

POULTRY & SEAFOOD MAINS

Chicken and Broccoli Stir-Fry

Preparation Time: 10 minutes
Cook Time: 15 minutes
Servings: 4

Ingredients

- 2 tablespoons sesame oil (or olive oil), divided
- 2 boneless, skinless chicken breasts, cubed
- 2 garlic cloves, minced
- 3 small carrots, thinly sliced
- 15 ounces frozen chopped broccoli florets, thawed
- 8 ounces sliced water chestnuts, drained and thoroughly rinsed
- 3 tablespoons balsamic vinegar, divided
- 2 teaspoons ground ginger

Directions

1. Heat ½ tablespoon of olive oil in a wok or large sauté pan over medium heat. Add the cubed chicken and cook until lightly browned and cooked through (about 5 to 7 minutes). Transfer chicken to a bowl, cover, and set aside.
2. Add 1½ tablespoons of olive oil to the pan, along with the garlic and carrots. Cook until the

carrots begin to soften (about 3 to 4 minutes). Add the thawed broccoli florets and water chestnuts along with 1 tablespoon of balsamic vinegar and cook for 3 to 4 minutes.

3. Add the remaining balsamic vinegar and ground ginger. Add the cooked chicken and stir until well combined.

4. Serve over brown rice, if desired.

Nutritional Values: Per Serving Total Calories: 189; Total Fat: 9g; Saturated Fat: 2g; Cholesterol: 33mg; Sodium: 68mg; Potassium: 228mg; Total Carbohydrates: 12g; Fiber: 3g; Sugars: 3g; Protein: 14g

Quick Chicken Fajitas

Preparation Time: 10 minutes
Cook Time: 15 minutes
Servings: 4

Ingredients

- Cooking spray
- 4 cups frozen bell pepper strips
- 2 cups onion, sliced
- 1 pound boneless, skinless chicken breast, cut into thin slices
- 1 teaspoon ground cumin
- 1 teaspoon chili powder
- 2 (10-ounce) cans no-salt diced tomatoes and green chilies (Ro-Tel brand)
- 8 (6-inch) whole-wheat flour tortillas, warmed

Directions

1. Spray a large skillet with cooking spray. Preheat skillet to medium-high heat. Add the bell peppers and onions and cook for 7 minutes or until tender, stirring occasionally. Remove from skillet and set aside.
2. Add chicken to skillet. Sprinkle with cumin and chili powder. Cook for 4 minutes until no longer pink and an instant-read thermometer registers 165°F.

3. Return peppers and onions to skillet; add drained tomatoes and green chilies. Cook for 2 minutes more or until hot.
4. Divide mixture evenly between tortillas and serve immediately.

Nutritional Values: Per Serving Total Calories: 424; Total Fat: 8g; Saturated Fat: 2g; Cholesterol: 65mg; Sodium: 622mg; Potassium: 138mg; Total Carbohydrates: 51g; Fiber: 26g; Sugars: 5g; Protein: 33g

Honey-Mustard Chicken

Preparation Time: 5 minutes
Cook Time: 15 minutes
Servings: 4

Ingredients

- ¼ cup honey
- ¼ cup yellow mustard
- ¼ cup Dijon mustard
- 1 tablespoon olive oil
- 1 pound boneless, skinless chicken breasts
- 3 cups broccoli florets
- ½ teaspoon freshly ground black pepper

Directions

1. To a medium bowl, add the honey, yellow mustard, and Dijon mustard. Whisk to combine. Taste to check for flavor balance, adding more honey and mustard if necessary. Set aside.
2. In a large skillet, add the oil and chicken.
Cook over medium-high heat for 3 to 5 minutes, then turn over and cook for an additional 3 to 5 minutes. Cooking time will vary depending on the thickness of the chicken. Chicken should be almost cooked through.

3. Evenly drizzle the honey mustard over the chicken and turn each piece over a few times to ensure both sides are evenly coated.

4. Add the broccoli and stir to combine, making sure the broccoli gets coated with honey mustard. Cover and cook over medium-low heat, allowing the broccoli to steam for about 3 to 5 minutes or until broccoli is crisp-tender and chicken is cooked through and an instant-read thermometer registers 165°F.

5. Serve immediately.

Nutritional Values: Per Serving Total Calories: 254; Total Fat: 8g; Saturated Fat: 2g; Cholesterol: 65mg; Sodium: 584mg; Potassium: 229mg; Total Carbohydrates: 21g; Fiber: 2g; Sugars: 17g; Protein: 27g

Grilled Chicken, Avocado, and Apple Salad

Preparation Time: 15 minutes
Cook Time: 8 minutes
Servings: 4

Ingredients

- Cooking spray
- 2 tablespoons olive oil
- 3 tablespoons balsamic vinegar
- 4 (4-ounce) skinless, boneless chicken-breast halves
- 8 cups mixed salad greens
- 1 cup diced peeled apple
- ¾ cup avocado, peeled and pitted
- *Optional:* 2 tablespoons freshly squeezed lime juice

Directions

1. Preheat grill to high heat. Apply cooking spray to the grill rack. If you don't have a grill, broil the chicken in an oven-safe skillet under the broiler element for 5 to 6 minutes.

2. Combine olive oil, balsamic vinegar, and lime juice (if using) in a small bowl. Place chicken on a large plate. Spoon 2 tablespoons of oil mixture over the chicken, reserving the rest for the salad

dressing. Turn chicken to coat and let stand for 5 minutes.

3. Place chicken on grill rack. Cook for 4 minutes on each side or until an instant-read thermometer registers 165°F. Remove and put on a plate. Cut crosswise into strips.

4. Arrange greens, apple, and avocado on 4 serving plates. Arrange chicken over greens. Drizzle reserved dressing over salads.

Nutritional Values: Per Serving Total Calories: 288; Total Fat: 16g; Saturated Fat: 3g; Cholesterol: 65mg; Sodium: 81mg; Potassium: 175mg; Total Carbohydrates: 8g; Fiber: 5g; Sugars: 4g; Protein: 27g

Turkey Cutlets with Herbs

Preparation Time: 5 minutes
Cook Time: 8 minutes
Servings: 4

Ingredients

- 2 tablespoons olive oil
- 2 lemons, sliced
- 1 package (approximately 1 pound) turkey breast cutlets (without antibiotics)
- ½ teaspoon garlic powder
- Freshly ground black pepper
- 4 cups baby spinach
- ½ cup water
- 2 teaspoons dried thyme

Directions

1. In a large skillet over medium-high heat, heat the oil.

2. Add about 6 lemon slices to the skillet.

3. Sprinkle the turkey-breast cutlets with garlic powder and black pepper. Place the turkey cutlets into the skillet and cook for about 3 minutes on each side until the turkey is no longer pink and is slightly browned at the edges. Remove from heat and divide turkey between 4 plates.

4. Add the spinach to the pan along with ½ cup of water and steam, stirring frequently for about 2 minutes. Remove the greens and lemons with tongs or a slotted spoon and divide between plates.
5. Serve topped with dried thyme.

Nutritional Values: Per Serving Total Calories: 204; Total Fat: 8g; Saturated Fat: 1g; Cholesterol: 70mg; Sodium: 92mg; Potassium: 82mg; Total Carbohydrates: 8g; Fiber: 4g; Sugars: 1g; Protein: 30g

Easy Roast Salmon with Roasted Asparagus

Preparation Time: 5 minutes
Cook Time: 15 minutes
Servings: 2

Ingredients

- 2 (5-ounce) salmon fillets with skin
- 2 teaspoons olive oil, plus extra for drizzling
- Salt
- Freshly ground black pepper
- 1 bunch asparagus, trimmed
- 1 teaspoon dried chives
- 1 teaspoon dried tarragon
- Fresh lemon wedges for serving

Directions

1. Preheat the oven to 425°F.

2. Rub salmon completely with 1 teaspoon of olive oil per fillet. Season with salt and pepper.

3. Place asparagus spears on a foil-lined baking sheet and lay the salmon fillets skin-side down on top. Put the pan in the upper third of oven and roast until fish is just cooked through (about 12 minutes). Roasting time will vary depending on the thickness of your salmon. Salmon should flake easily with a fork when it's ready and an instant-read thermometer should register 145°F.

4. When cooked, remove from the oven, cut fillets in half crosswise, then lift flesh from skin with a metal spatula and transfer to a plate. Discard the skin. Drizzle salmon with oil, sprinkle with herbs and serve with lemon wedges and roasted asparagus spears.

Nutritional Values: Per Serving Total Calories: 353; Total Fat: 22g; Saturated Fat: 4g; Cholesterol: 88mg; Sodium: 90mg; Potassium: 304mg; Total Carbohydrates: 5g; Fiber: 2g; Sugars: 0g; Protein: 34g

Shrimp Pasta Primavera

Preparation Time: 5 minutes
Cook Time: 15 minutes
Servings: 2

Ingredients

- 2 tablespoons olive oil
- 1 tablespoon garlic, minced
- 2 cups assorted fresh vegetables, chopped coarsely (zucchini, broccoli, asparagus or whatever you prefer)
- 4 ounces frozen shrimp, cooked, peeled, and deveined
- Salt
- Freshly ground black pepper
- Juice of ½ lemon
- 4 ounces whole-wheat angel-hair pasta, cooked per package instructions
- 2 tablespoons grated Parmesan cheese

Directions

1. Heat the oil in a large nonstick skillet over medium heat. Add the garlic and sauté for 1 minute.
2. Add vegetables and sauté until crisp-tender (about 3 to 4 minutes).

3. Add the shrimp and sauté until just heated through. Season lightly with salt and pepper and squeeze lemon juice over the shrimp and vegetables. Continue to cook for about 2 minutes until the juices have been reduced by about half. Remove from heat.

4. Toss shrimp and vegetables with pasta. Serve topped with Parmesan cheese.

Nutritional Values: Per Serving Total Calories: 439; Total Fat: 17g; Saturated Fat: 3g; Cholesterol: 105mg; Sodium: 286mg; Potassium: 481mg; Total Carbohydrates: 50g; Fiber: 8g; Sugars: 5g; Protein: 23g

Cilantro-Lime Tilapia Tacos

Preparation Time: 10 minutes
Cook Time: 10 minutes
Servings: 4

Ingredients

- 1 teaspoon olive oil
- 1 pound tilapia fillets, rinsed and dried
- 3 cups diced tomatoes
- ½ cup fresh cilantro, chopped, plus additional for serving
- 3 tablespoons freshly squeezed lime juice
- Salt
- Freshly ground black pepper
- 8 (5-inch) white corn tortillas
- 1 avocado sliced into 8 wedges
- *Optional:* lime wedges and fat-free sour cream for serving

Directions

1. Heat the oil in a large skillet, add the tilapia and cook until the flesh starts to flake (about 5 minutes per side).
2. Add the tomatoes, cilantro, and lime juice. Sauté over medium-high heat for about 5 minutes, breaking up the fish and mixing well. Season to taste with salt and pepper.

3. Heat tortillas in a skillet for a few minutes on each side to warm.

4. Serve ¼ cup of fish mixture on each warmed tortilla with two slices of avocado.

5. Serve immediately with optional toppings.

Nutritional Values: Per Serving Total Calories: 286; Total Fat: 12g; Saturated Fat: 2g; Cholesterol: 55mg; Sodium: 117mg; Potassium: 860mg; Total Carbohydrates: 22g; Fiber: 4g; Sugars: 0g; Protein: 28g

Lemon-Parsley Baked Flounder and Brussels Sprouts

Preparation Time: 10 minutes
Cook Time: 15 minutes
Servings: 2

Ingredients

- 14 Brussels sprouts
- 2 tablespoons olive oil, divided
- 3 tablespoons freshly squeezed lemon juice
- 1 tablespoon minced fresh garlic
- ¼ teaspoon dried dill
- 2 (6-ounce) flounder fillets
- Salt
- Freshly ground black pepper

Directions

1. Preheat the oven to 400°F. Rinse the Brussels sprouts and pat them dry. Cut their stem ends off, cut sprouts in half and place them on a foil-lined baking pan. Drizzle with 1 tablespoon olive oil and toss to coat.

2. In a small bowl, stir together 1 tablespoon olive oil, lemon juice, garlic, and dill.

3. Rinse flounder fillets and pat dry. Season lightly with salt and pepper. Place in a baking dish and

evenly drizzle oil-and-herb mixture over flounder fillets.

4. Bake for 10 to 11 minutes or until the fish flakes easily when tested with a fork. The Brussels sprouts should be lightly browned and also pierce easily with a fork.

5. Divide the flounder and Brussels sprouts between serving plates.

Nutritional Values: Per Serving Total Calories: 319; Total Fat: 17g; Saturated Fat: 2g; Cholesterol: 98mg; Sodium: 529mg; Potassium: 538mg; Total Carbohydrates: 13g; Fiber: 5g; Sugars: 3g; Protein: 33g

Pan-Seared Scallops

Preparation Time: 5 minutes
Cook Time: 6 minutes
Servings: 4

Ingredients

- 2 cups chopped tomato
- ½ cup chopped fresh basil
- ¼ teaspoon freshly ground black pepper, divided
- 2 tablespoons olive oil, divided
- 1½ pounds sea scallops
- ⅛ teaspoon salt
- 1 cup fresh corn kernels
- 1 cup zucchini, diced

Directions

1. In a medium bowl, combine tomato, basil, and ⅛ teaspoon black pepper. Toss gently.
2. Heat a large skillet over high heat. Add 1 tablespoon of olive oil to the pan, swirling to coat. Pat scallops dry with paper towels. Sprinkle with salt and remaining black pepper. Add scallops to the pan, cook for 2 minutes or until browned. Turn scallops and cook for 2 minutes more or until browned. Remove scallops from the pan and keep warm.

3. Heat the remaining olive oil in the pan. Add corn and zucchini to the pan. Sauté for 2 minutes or until lightly browned. Add to tomato mixture and toss gently.

4. Serve scallops with a spinach salad, if desired.

Nutritional Values: Per Serving Total Calories: 221; Total Fat: 9g; Saturated Fat: 1g; Cholesterol: 35mg; Sodium: 214mg; Potassium: 444mg; Total Carbohydrates: 17g; Fiber: 3g; Sugars: 5g; Protein: 20g

Baked Cod Packets with Broccoli and Squash

Preparation Time: 10 minutes
Cook Time: 20 minutes
Servings: 4

Ingredients

- 2 cups summer squash, sliced
- 2 cups small broccoli florets
- 4 garlic cloves, minced
- 2 tablespoons olive oil
- Salt
- Freshly ground black pepper
- 4 (4-ounce) cod fillets
- 4 teaspoons dried thyme
- Juice of 1 lemon

Directions

1. Preheat the oven to 400°F. Cut aluminum foil into 4, 12-inch squares and arrange them on a work surface. Fold each piece in half to form a crease down the middle. Spray the foil with cooking spray.

2. Divide squash between the squares, arranging it just to the right of each crease. Top squash with broccoli and garlic. Drizzle with olive oil and sprinkle with salt and pepper.

3. Arrange 1 fillet on top of each pile of vegetables and then season fillets with salt and pepper. Top each fillet with 1 teaspoon of dried thyme.

4. Drizzle lemon juice over the fillets. Wrap each square of foil to form a sealed pouch. Transfer pouches to a baking sheet and bake until the fish is cooked through (about 20 minutes).

5. Set aside to rest for 3 to 4 minutes. Then cut pouches open, being careful of the steam. Serve immediately.

Nutritional Values: Per Serving Total Calories: 184; Total Fat: 8g; Saturated Fat: 1g; Cholesterol: 40mg; Sodium: 95mg; Potassium: 397mg; Total Carbohydrates: 8g; Fiber: 3g; Sugars: 2g; Protein: 22g

Garlic Salmon and Snap Peas In Foil

Preparation Time: 5 minutes
Cook Time: 15 minutes
Servings: 2

Ingredients

- Cooking spray
- 2 (4-ounce) skinless salmon fillets
- 2 cups sugar snap peas, divided
- 2 garlic cloves, minced and divided
- Juice of 1 lemon, divided
- Salt
- Freshly ground black pepper

Directions

1. Preheat the oven to 450°F.
2. Cut 2 large squares of aluminum foil, each about 12-by-18 inches. Spray the center of each foil sheet with cooking spray.
3. Place 1 salmon fillet in the center of each sheet, top with 1 cup of sugar snap peas, 1 clove minced garlic, and drizzle with lemon juice. Sprinkle with salt and pepper if desired.
4. Bring up the sides of the foil and fold the top over twice.
5. Seal ends, leaving room for air to circulate inside the packet.

6. Place packets on a baking sheet.

Cook Time: bake for 15 to 18 minutes, or until salmon is opaque.

7. Use caution when opening the packets as the steam will be very hot. Serve with lemon wedges on the side, if desired.

Nutritional Values: Per Serving Total Calories: 211; Total Fat: 5g; Saturated Fat: 1g; Cholesterol: 50mg; Sodium: 86mg; Potassium: 41mg; Total Carbohydrates: 14g; Fiber: 3g; Sugars: 5g; Protein: 26g

Southwestern Chicken and Pasta

Preparation Time: 10 minutes
Cooking Time: 10 minutes
Servings: 2

Ingredients

- 1 cup uncooked whole-wheat rigatoni
- 2 boneless, skinless chicken breasts, 4 ounces each, cut into cubes
- 1/4 cup salsa
- 1 1/2 cups canned unsalted tomato sauce
- 1/8 teaspoon garlic powder
- 1 teaspoon cumin
- 1/2 teaspoon chili powder
- 1/2 cup canned black beans, rinsed and drained
- 1/2 cup fresh or canned corn
- 1/4 cup shredded Monterey Jack and Colby cheese

Directions

1. Fill a pot with water up to ¾ full and boil it.
2. Add pasta to water and cook until it is al dente. Drain the pasta while rinsing under cold water.
3. Preheat a skillet with cooking oil, then cook the chicken for 10 minutes until golden on both sides.
4. Add tomato sauce, salsa, cumin, garlic powder, black beans, corn, and chili powder.

5. Stir while cooking the mixture for a few minutes. Add in pasta.

6. Serve with 2 tablespoons cheese on top.

7. Enjoy.

Nutritional Values: Per Serving Calories 245 Total Fat 16.3 G Saturated Fat 4.9 G Cholesterol 114 Mg Sodium 515 Mg Total Carbohydrates 19.3 G Fiber 0.1 G Sugar 18.2 G Protein 33.3 G

Buffalo Chicken Salad Wrap

Preparation Time: 10 minutes
Cooking Time: 10 minutes
Servings: 4

Ingredients:

- 3-4 ounces chicken breasts
- 2 whole chipotle peppers
- 1/4 cup white wine vinegar
- 1/4 cup low-calorie mayonnaise
- 2 stalks celery, diced
- 2 carrots, cut into matchsticks
- 1 small yellow onion, diced (about 1/2 cup)
- 1/2 cup thinly sliced rutabaga or another root vegetable
- 4 ounces spinach, cut into strips
- 2 whole-grain tortillas (12-inch diameter)

Directions

1. Set the oven or a grill to heat at 375°F. Bake the chicken for 10 minutes per side.
2. Blend chipotle peppers with mayonnaise and wine vinegar in the blender.
3. Dice the baked chicken into cubes or small chunks.
4. Mix the chipotle mixture with all the ingredients except tortillas and spinach.

5. Spread 2 ounces of spinach over the tortilla and scoop the stuffing on top.
6. Wrap the tortilla and cut it into the half.
7. Serve.

Nutritional Values: Per Serving Calories 300 Total Fat 16.4 g; Saturated Fat 9.1 g; Cholesterol 143 mg; Sodium 471 mg; Total Carbohydrates 8.7 g; Fiber 0.7 g; Sugar 0.3 g; Protein 38.5 g

Chicken Sliders

Preparation Time: 10 minutes
Cooking Time: 10 minutes
Servings: 4

Ingredients:

- 10 ounces ground chicken breast
- 1 tablespoon black pepper
- 1 tablespoon minced garlic
- 1 tablespoon balsamic vinegar
- 1/2 cup minced onion
- 1 fresh chili pepper, minced
- 1 tablespoon fennel seed, crushed
- 4 whole-wheat mini buns
- 4 lettuce leaves
- 4 tomato slices

Directions

1. Combine all the ingredients except the wheat buns, tomato, and lettuce.
2. Mix well and refrigerate the mixture for 1 hour.
3. Divide the mixture into 4 patties.
4. Broil the patties on a greased baking sheet until golden brown.
5. Place the chicken patties in the whole wheat buns along with lettuce and tomato.
6. Serve.

Nutritional Values: Per Serving Calories 224; Total Fat 4.5 g; Saturated Fat 3.8 g; Cholesterol 183 mg; Sodium 212 mg; Total Carbohydrates 10.2 g; Fiber 1.6 g; Sugar 0.5 g; Protein 67.4 g

BEEF & PORK MAINS

Mustard-Crusted Pork Tenderloin

Preparation Time: 15 minutes
Cook Time: 15 minutes
Servings: 4

Ingredients

- 3 tablespoons Dijon mustard
- 3 tablespoons honey
- 1 teaspoon dried rosemary
- 1 tablespoon olive oil
- 1 pound pork tenderloin
- Salt
- Freshly ground black pepper

Directions

1. Preheat the oven to 425°F with the rack set in the middle. In a small bowl, combine the Dijon mustard, honey, and rosemary. Stir to combine and set aside.
2. Preheat an oven-safe skillet over high heat and add the olive oil. While it is heating up, pat pork loin dry with a paper towel and season lightly with salt and pepper on all sides. When the skillet is hot, sear the pork loin on all sides until golden brown (about 3 minutes per side). Remove from

the heat and spread honey-mustard mixture evenly to coat the pork loin.

3. Place the skillet in the oven and cook the pork loin for 15 minutes, or until an instant-read thermometer registers 145°F.

4. Remove from the oven and allow to rest for 3 minutes. Slice the pork into ½-inch slices and serve.

Nutritional Values: Per Serving Total Calories: 220; Total Fat: 9g; Saturated Fat: 3g; Cholesterol: 45mg; Sodium: 307mg; Potassium: 11mg; Total Carbohydrates: 14g; Fiber: 0g; Sugars: 13g; Protein: 19g

Pork Medallions with Spring Succotash

Preparation Time: 10 minutes
Cook Time: 20 minutes
Servings: 4

Ingredients

- 1 pound pork tenderloin, trimmed and cut into 1-inch-thick slices
- 2 teaspoons minced garlic
- 1 teaspoon dried rosemary
- 1½ tablespoons olive oil, divided
- 1 cup low-sodium chicken stock
- 1 cup carrots, halved and thinly sliced
- 3 tablespoons water
- ½ teaspoon freshly ground black pepper
- 2 cups frozen lima beans, thawed
- 1 cup frozen spinach, thawed

Directions

1. Gently pound pork slices to ½-inch-thick medallions with a meat mallet or the heel of your hand.
2. Combine garlic and rosemary in a small bowl.
3. Heat a large skillet over medium heat. Add 1 tablespoon of olive oil and swirl to coat. Add the pork to the pan and cook for 4 minutes without

turning. Turn and cook for 3 minutes or until done. Remove pork from pan and keep warm.

4. Add garlic mixture; sauté for 1 minute or until fragrant. Add chicken stock and cook for 30 seconds or until reduced to ½ cup. Remove pan from heat.

5. Heat a second large nonstick skillet over medium heat. Add remaining olive oil and swirl to coat. Add carrots and cook for 2 minutes. Stir in water and black pepper. Cover and cook for 2 minutes until carrots are crisp-tender. Stir in lima beans and spinach, Cook for 3 minutes or until thoroughly heated.

6. Divide vegetable mixture among 4 plates. Top each serving with pork and sauce.

Nutritional Values: Per Serving Total Calories: 317; Total Fat: 11g; Saturated Fat: 3g; Cholesterol: 45mg; Sodium: 150mg; Potassium: 626mg; Total Carbohydrates: 28g; Fiber: 8g; Sugars: 2g; Protein: 28g

Pork Salad with Walnuts and Peaches

Preparation Time: 15 minutes
Cook Time: 10 minutes
Servings: 4

Ingredients

- 1 tablespoon olive oil
- 1 pound pork tenderloin, cut into 1-inch cubes
- 1 (10-ounce) bag fresh spinach leaves
- 1 peach, pitted and sliced
- ¼ cup walnuts
- Balsamic vinegar

Directions

1. Heat the olive oil in a large nonstick skillet over medium-high heat. Add the pork and cook until it is browned on the outside and cooked through (3 to 4 minutes per side). Remove from heat and set aside.
2. Make a bed of spinach on each individual serving plate. Arrange peach slices over the spinach. Top with the cooked pork and sprinkle with walnuts. Drizzle balsamic vinegar over the salad.
3. Enjoy immediately.

Nutritional Values: Per Serving Total Calories: 230; Total Fat: 14g; Saturated Fat: 3g; Cholesterol: 45mg; Sodium: 69mg; Potassium: 81mg; Total Carbohydrates: 6g; Fiber: 2g; Sugars: 2g; Protein: 21g

Pork, White Bean, and Spinach Soup

Preparation Time: 10 minutes
Cook Time: 15 minutes
Servings: 4

Ingredients

- 1 tablespoon olive oil
- 8 ounces pork tenderloin or boneless pork chops, cut into 1-inch cubes
- Salt
- 4 garlic cloves, minced
- 2 teaspoons paprika
- 1 (14.5-ounce) can diced salt-free tomatoes
- 4 cups low-sodium chicken broth
- 1 bunch spinach, ribs removed and chopped, about 8 cups, lightly packed
- 2 (15-ounce) cans white beans, drained and rinsed

Directions

1. Heat the oil in a Dutch oven or heavy-bottom pot over medium-high heat. Season pork with a pinch of salt. When the pan is hot, add pork and cook, stirring occasionally, for about 2 minutes, or long enough to encourage a good sear and brown sides. Transfer to a plate.

2. In the same pot, add the garlic and paprika. Cook, stirring often, until fragrant (about 30 seconds). Add tomatoes and increase heat to high and stir to scrape down any browned bits. Add broth and bring to a boil.

3. Add spinach until it just wilts (about 2 to 3 minutes). Reduce heat to maintain a simmer, stir in the beans, reserved pork, and any accumulated juices; simmer until the beans and pork are heated through (about 2 minutes).

4. Serve immediately.

Nutritional Values: Per Serving Total Calories: 327; Total Fat: 8g; Saturated Fat: 2g; Cholesterol: 22mg; Sodium: 389mg; Potassium: 511mg; Total Carbohydrates: 41g; Fiber: 15g; Sugars: 5g; Protein: 26g

Orange-Beef Stir-Fry

Preparation Time: 10 minutes
Cook Time: 10 minutes
Servings: 2

Ingredients

- 1 tablespoon cornstarch
- ¼ cup cold water
- ¼ cup orange juice
- 1 tablespoon reduced-sodium soy sauce
- ½ pound boneless beef sirloin steak, cut into thin strips
- 2 teaspoons olive oil, divided
- 3 cups frozen stir-fry vegetable blend
- 1 garlic clove, minced

Directions

1. In a small bowl, combine the cornstarch, cold water, orange juice, and soy sauce until smooth. Set aside.
2. In a large skillet or wok, stir-fry beef in 1 teaspoon of olive oil for 3 to 4 minutes or until no longer pink. Remove with a slotted spoon and keep warm.
3. Stir-fry the vegetable blend and garlic in the remaining oil for 3 minutes. Stir cornstarch mixture and add to the pan. Bring to a boil. Cook

stirring constantly, for 2 minutes or until thickened. Add the beef and heat through.

Nutritional Values: Per Serving Total Calories: 268; Total Fat: 10g; Saturated Fat: 3g; Cholesterol: 65mg; Sodium: 376mg; Potassium: 65mg; Total Carbohydrates: 8g; Fiber: 3g; Sugars: 8g; Protein: 26g

Steak Tacos

Preparation Time: 15 minutes
Cook Time: 13 minutes
Servings: 4

Ingredients

- 1 pound beef flank (or round) steak
- 1 teaspoon chili powder
- 1 teaspoon olive oil
- 1 green bell pepper, cored and coarsely chopped
- 1 red onion, coarsely chopped
- 8 (6-inch) corn tortillas, warm
- 2 tablespoons freshly squeezed lime juice
- *Optional for serving:* 1 avocado, sliced, and coarsely chopped cilantro

Directions

1. Rub the steak with chili powder (and salt and pepper, if desired).
2. Heat olive oil in a large skillet over medium-high heat.
3. Add steak and cook for 6 to 8 minutes on each side or until it is done. Remove from heat.
4. Place steak on a plate and cover with aluminum foil. Let rest for 5 minutes.
5. Add the bell pepper and onion to skillet. Cook on medium heat, stirring frequently, for 3 to 5

minutes or until onion is translucent. Remove from heat.

6. Cut steak against the grain into thin slices.

7. Top tortillas evenly with beef, onion mixture, and lime juice. Garnish with avocado and cilantro, if desired.

8. Serve immediately.

Nutritional Values: Per Serving Total Calories: 358; Total Fat: 12g; Saturated Fat: 4g; Cholesterol: 40mg; Sodium: 139mg; Potassium: 503mg; Total Carbohydrates: 34g; Fiber: 2g; Sugars: 0g; Protein: 28g

Beef-and-Bean Chili

Preparation Time: 5 minutes
Cook Time: 20 minutes
Servings: 4

Ingredients

- 1 pound lean or extra-lean ground beef
- 1 yellow onion, diced
- 3 (15-ounce) cans salt-free diced tomatoes with green chilies (Ro-Tel brand)
- 2 (15-ounce) cans beans, drained and rinsed (whatever you desire: black, red, pinto, kidney, etc.)
- 2 tablespoons chili powder
- *Optional:* 1 (10-ounce) package frozen spinach

Directions

1. In a large stockpot, cook the beef over medium-high heat until browned, stirring frequently. Using a slotted spoon, transfer the cooked beef to a separate plate and set aside. Reserve 1 tablespoon of grease in the stockpot and discard the rest.
2. Add the onion to the stockpot and sauté for 4 to 5 minutes until soft.
3. Add the tomatoes with green chilies, beans, chili powder, and cooked beef to the stockpot. Stir to

combine. Bring to a boil and then reduce heat to medium-low. Cover and simmer for 10 minutes.
4. Serve immediately.

Nutritional Values: Per Serving Total Calories: 429; Total Fat: 10g; Saturated Fat: 3g; Cholesterol: 65mg; Sodium: 322mg; Potassium: 816mg; Total Carbohydrates: 47g; Fiber: 16g; Sugars: 0g; Protein: 38g

Asian Pork Tenderloin

Preparation Time: 10 minutes
Cooking Time: 15 minutes
Servings: 4

Ingredients:

- 2 tablespoons sesame seeds
- 1 teaspoon ground coriander
- 1/8 teaspoon cayenne pepper
- 1/8 teaspoon celery seed
- 1/2 teaspoon minced onion
- 1/4 teaspoon ground cumin
- 1/8 teaspoon ground cinnamon
- 1 tablespoon sesame oil
- 1-pound pork tenderloin, sliced into 4 4-ounce portions

Directions

1. Set the oven to heat at 400°F. Grease a baking dish with cooking oil.
2. Toast the sesame seeds in a dry frying pan until golden brown.
3. Transfer the sesame seeds to a bowl and set it aside.
4. Combine coriander with celery seed, cinnamon, toasted sesame seeds, cumin, sesame oil, and minced onion in a bowl.

5. Place the pork tenderloin in a baking dish and rub them with pepper mixture.
6. Bake them for 15 minutes.
7. Serve.

Nutritional Values: Calories 248; Total Fat 13.8 g; Saturated Fat 4.9 g; Cholesterol 125 mg; Sodium 587 mg; Total Carbohydrates 1.1 g; Fiber 3.1g; Sugar 0.2 g; Protein 55.9 g

Curried Pork Tenderloin in Apple Cider

Preparation Time: 6 minutes
Cooking Time: 15 minutes
Servings: 6

Ingredients

- 16 ounces pork tenderloin, cut into 6 pieces
- 1 1/2 tablespoons curry powder
- 1 tablespoon extra-virgin olive oil
- 2 medium yellow onions, chopped (about 2 cups)
- 2 cups apple cider, divided
- 1 tart apple, peeled, seeded, and chopped into chunks
- 1 tablespoon cornstarch

Directions

1. Rub the pork tenderloin with curry powder and let it rest for 15 minutes.
2. Preheat a skillet with olive oil on medium heat.
3. Sear the tenderloin for 10 minutes per side and then transfer it to a plate.
4. Add onions to the same skillet and sauté until golden and soft.
5. Stir in 1 ½ cups apple cider and cook until it is reduced to half.

6. Add chopped apples, remaining apple cider, and cornstarch.

7. Stir and then cook the mixture for 2 minutes until it thickens.

8. Return the tenderloin to the sauce.

9. Let it cook for 5 minutes in the sauce.

10. Serve and enjoy.

Nutritional Values: Calories 244; Total Fat 14.8 g; Saturated Fat 3.1 g; Cholesterol 101 mg; Sodium 372 mg; Total Carbohydrates 19.4 g; Fiber 1.3 g; Sugar 0.3 g; Protein 10.2 g

New York Strip Steak

Preparation Time: 15 minutes
Cooking Time: 20 minutes
Servings: 2

Ingredients:

- 2 New York strip steaks, 4 ounces each, trimmed of all visible fat
- 1 teaspoon trans-free margarine
- 3 garlic cloves, chopped
- 2 ounces sliced shiitake mushrooms
- 2 ounces button mushrooms
- 1/4 teaspoon thyme
- 1/4 teaspoon rosemary
- 1/4 cup whiskey

Directions

1. Preheat a charcoal grill or broiler. Grease the racks with cooking spray.
2. Place the greased rack about 4 inches away from the heat source.
3. Grill the steaks on the preheated grill for 10 minutes per side.
4. Sauté garlic with mushrooms, rosemary, and thyme in a greased skillet.
5. Cook for 2 minutes and then stir in whiskey after removing the pan from the heat.

6. Pour this sauce over steaks.
7. Serve.

Nutritional Values: Calories 330; Total Fat 9.8 g; Saturated Fat 3.4 g; Cholesterol 22 mg; Sodium 671 mg; Total Carbohydrates 21.1 g; Fiber 3.1 g; Sugar 0.3 g; Protein 44 g

Pork Medallions with Herbs de Provence

Preparation Time: 10 minutes
Cooking Time: 20 minutes
Servings: 4

Ingredients

- 8 ounces pork tenderloin, trimmed of visible fat and cut crosswise into 6 pieces
- Freshly ground black pepper, to taste
- 1/2 teaspoon herbs de Provence
- 1/4 cup dry white wine

Directions

1. Season the pork with black pepper and place the meat between sheets of parchment paper.
2. Punch the pork pieces with a mallet into ¼ inch thickness.
3. Sear the seasoned pork in a greased skillet for 3 minutes per side.
4. Remove it from the pan and drizzle with herbs de Provence.
5. Transfer the pork to the serving plate.
6. Add wine to the same skillet and scrape off the brown bits while stirring.
7. Pour this wine over the medallions.
8. Serve warm.

Nutritional Values: Calories 120; Total Fat 24 g; Saturated Fat 18.5 g; Cholesterol 49 mg; Sodium 647 mg; Total Carbohydrates 26.4 g; Fiber 1.5 g; Sugar 1.1 g; Protein 23.4 g

SNACKS, SIDES & DESSERTS

Southwestern Bean-and-Pepper Salad

Preparation Time: 6 minutes
Servings: 4

Ingredients

- 1 (15-ounce) can pinto beans, drained and rinsed
- 2 bell peppers, cored and chopped
- 1 cup corn kernels (cut from 1 to 2 ears or frozen and thawed)
- Salt
- Freshly ground black pepper
- Juice of 2 limes
- 1 tablespoon olive oil
- 1 avocado, chopped

Directions

1. In a large bowl, combine beans, peppers, corn, salt, and pepper. Squeeze fresh lime juice to taste and stir in olive oil. Let the mixture stand in the refrigerator for 30 minutes.
2. Add avocado just before serving.

Nutritional Values: Per Serving Total Calories: 245; Total Fat: 11g; Saturated Fat: 2g; Cholesterol: 0mg; Sodium: 97mg; Potassium: 380mg; Total Carbohydrates: 32g; Fiber: 10g; Sugars: 4g; Protein: 8g

Cauliflower Mashed "Potatoes"

Preparation Time: 10 minutes
Cook Time: 10 minutes
Servings: 4

Ingredients

- 16 cups water (enough to cover cauliflower)
- 1 head cauliflower (about 3 pounds), trimmed and cut into florets
- 4 garlic cloves
- 1 tablespoon olive oil
- ¼ teaspoon salt
- ⅛ teaspoon freshly ground black pepper
- 2 teaspoons dried parsley

Directions

1. Bring a large pot of water to a boil. Add the cauliflower and garlic. Cook for about 10 minutes or until the cauliflower is fork-tender. Drain, return it back to the hot pan and let it stand for 2 to 3 minutes with the lid on.
2. Transfer the cauliflower and garlic to a food processor or blender. Add the olive oil, salt, and pepper, and purée until smooth.
3. Taste and adjust the salt and pepper. Remove to a serving bowl and add the parsley and mix until combined.

4. Garnish with additional olive oil, if desired.
5. Serve immediately.

Nutritional Values: Per Serving Total Calories: 87; Total Fat: 4g; Saturated Fat: 1g; Cholesterol: 0mg; Sodium: 210mg; Potassium: 654mg; Total Carbohydrates: 12g; Fiber: 5g; Sugars: 0g; Protein: 4g

Roasted Brussels Sprouts

Preparation Time: 5 minutes
Cook Time: 20 minutes
Servings: 4

Ingredients

- 1½ pounds Brussels sprouts, trimmed and halved
- 2 tablespoons olive oil
- ¼ teaspoon salt
- ½ teaspoon freshly ground black pepper

Directions

1. Preheat the oven to 400°F.
2. Combine the Brussels sprouts and olive oil in a large mixing bowl and toss until they are evenly coated.
3. Turn the Brussels sprouts out onto a large baking sheet and flip them over so they are cut-side down with the flat part touching the baking sheet. Sprinkle with salt and pepper.
4. Bake for 20 minutes or until the Brussels sprouts are lightly charred and crisp on the outside and toasted on the bottom. The outer leaves should be dark.
5. Serve immediately.

Nutritional Values: Per Serving Total Calories: 134; Total Fat: 8g; Saturated Fat: 1g; Cholesterol: 0mg; Sodium: 189mg; Potassium: 665mg; Total Carbohydrates: 15g; Fiber: 7g; Sugars: 4g; Protein: 6g

Broccoli with Garlic and Lemon

Preparation Time: 2 minutes
Cook Time: 4 minutes
Servings: 4

Ingredients

- 1 cup water
- 4 cups broccoli florets
- 1 teaspoon olive oil
- 1 tablespoon minced garlic
- 1 teaspoon lemon zest
- Salt
- Freshly ground black pepper

Directions

1. In a small saucepan, bring 1 cup of water to a boil. Add the broccoli to the boiling water and cook for 2 to 3 minutes or until tender, being careful not to overcook. The broccoli should retain its bright-green color. Drain the water from the broccoli.

2. In a small sauté pan over medium-high heat, add the olive oil. Add the garlic and sauté for 30 seconds. Add the broccoli, lemon zest, salt, and pepper. Combine well and serve.

Nutritional Values: Per Serving Total Calories: 38; Total Fat: 1g; Saturated Fat: 0g; Cholesterol: 0mg; Sodium: 24mg; Potassium: 295mg; Total Carbohydrates: 5g; Fiber: 3g; Sugars: 0g; Protein: 3g

Brown-Rice Pilaf

Preparation Time: 5 minutes
Cook Time: 10 minutes
Servings: 4

Ingredients

- 1 cup low-sodium vegetable broth
- ½ tablespoon olive oil
- 1 clove garlic, minced
- 1 scallion, thinly sliced
- 1 tablespoon minced onion flakes
- 1 cup instant brown rice
- ⅛ teaspoon freshly ground black pepper

Directions

1. Mix the vegetable broth, olive oil, garlic, scallion, and minced onion flakes in a saucepan and bring to a boil.
2. Add rice and return mixture to boil. Reduce heat and simmer for 10 minutes.
3. Remove from heat and let stand for 5 minutes.
4. Fluff with a fork and season with black pepper.

Nutritional Values: Per Serving Total Calories: 100; Total Fat: 2g; Saturated Fat: 0g; Cholesterol: 0mg; Sodium: 35mg; Potassium: 24mg; Total Carbohydrates: 19g; Fiber: 2g; Sugars: 1g; Protein: 2g

Chunky Black-Bean Dip

Preparation Time: 5 minutes
Servings: 6-8

Ingredients

- 1 (15-ounce) can black beans, drained, with liquid reserved
- ½ (7-ounce) can chipotle peppers in adobo sauce
- ¼ cup plain Greek yogurt
- Freshly ground black pepper

Directions

1. Combine beans, peppers, and yogurt in a food processor or blender and process until smooth. Add some of the bean liquid, 1 tablespoon at a time, for a thinner consistency.
2. Season to taste with black pepper.
3. Serve.

Nutritional Values: Per ⅓-Cup Serving Total Calories: 70; Total Fat: 1g; Saturated Fat: 0g; Cholesterol: 0mg; Sodium: 159mg; Potassium: 21mg; Total Carbohydrates: 11g; Fiber: 4g; Sugars: 0g; Protein: 5g

Classic Hummus

Preparation Time: 5 minutes
Servings: 6-8

Ingredients

- 1 (15-ounce) can chickpeas, drained and rinsed
- 3 tablespoons sesame tahini
- 2 tablespoons olive oil
- 3 garlic cloves, chopped
- Juice of 1 lemon
- Salt
- Freshly ground black pepper

Directions

1. In a food processor or blender, combine all the ingredients until smooth, but thick. Add water if necessary to produce a smoother hummus.
2. Store covered for up to 5 days.

Nutritional Values: Per ⅓-Cup Serving Total Calories: 147; Total Fat: 10g; Saturated Fat: 1g; Cholesterol: 0mg; Sodium: 64mg; Potassium: 16mg; Total Carbohydrates: 11g; Fiber: 4g; Sugars: 0g; Protein: 6g

Crispy Potato Skins

Preparation Time: 2 minutes
Cook Time: 19 minutes
Servings: 2

Ingredients

- 2 russet potatoes
- Cooking spray
- 1 teaspoon dried rosemary
- ⅛ teaspoon freshly ground black pepper

Directions

1. Preheat the oven to 375°F.
2. Wash the potatoes and pierce several times with a fork. Place on a plate. Cook on full power in the microwave for 5 minutes. Turn potatoes over and continue to cook for 3 to 4 minutes more, or until soft.
3. Carefully—the potatoes will be very hot—cut the potatoes in half and scoop out the pulp, leaving about ⅛ inch of potato flesh attached to the skin. Save the pulp for another use.
4. Spray the inside of each potato with cooking spray. Press in the rosemary and pepper. Place the skins on a baking sheet and bake in preheated oven for 5 to 10 minutes until slightly browned and crispy.

5. Serve immediately.

Nutritional Values: Per Serving Total Calories: 114; Total Fat: 0g; Saturated Fat: 0g; Cholesterol: 0mg; Sodium: 0mg; Potassium: 635mg; Total Carbohydrates: 27g; Fiber: 2g; Sugars: 1g; Protein: 3g

Carrot-Cake Smoothie

Preparation Time: 5 minutes
Servings: 2

Ingredients

- 1 frozen banana, peeled and diced
- 1 cup carrots, diced (peeled if preferred)
- 1 cup nonfat or low-fat milk
- ½ cup nonfat or low-fat vanilla Greek yogurt
- ½ cup ice
- ¼ cup diced pineapple, frozen
- ½ teaspoon ground cinnamon
- Pinch nutmeg
- *Optional toppings:* chopped walnuts, grated carrots

Directions

1. Add all of the ingredients to a blender and process until smooth and creamy.
2. Serve immediately with optional toppings as desired.

Nutritional Values: Per Serving Total Calories: 180; Total Fat: 1g; Saturated Fat: 0g; Cholesterol: 5mg; Sodium: 114mg; Potassium: 682mg; Total Carbohydrates: 36g; Fiber: 4g; Sugars: 25g; Protein: 10g

Chocolate Cake in a Mug

Preparation Time: 5 minutes
Cook Time: 1 minute
Servings: 1

Ingredients

- 3 tablespoons white whole-wheat flour
- 2 tablespoons unsweetened cocoa powder
- 2 teaspoons sugar
- ⅛ teaspoon baking powder
- 1 egg white
- ½ teaspoon olive oil
- 3 tablespoons nonfat or low-fat milk
- ½ teaspoon vanilla extract
- Cooking spray

Directions

1. Place the flour, cocoa, sugar, and baking powder in a small bowl and whisk until combined. Then add in the egg white, olive oil, milk, and vanilla extract. Mix to combine.
2. Spray a mug with cooking spray and pour batter into mug. Microwave on high for 60 seconds or until set.
3. Serve.

Nutritional Values: Per Serving Total Calories: 217; Total Fat: 4g; Saturated Fat: 1g; Cholesterol: 1mg; Sodium: 139mg; Potassium: 244mg; Total Carbohydrates: 35g; Fiber: 7g; Sugars: 12g; Protein: 11g

Peanut Butter Banana "Ice Cream"

Preparation Time: 10 minutes
Servings: 4

Ingredients

- 4 bananas, very ripe
- 2 tablespoons peanut butter

Directions

1. Peel bananas and slice into ½-inch disks. Arrange banana slices on a large plate or baking sheet. Freeze for 1 to 2 hours.
2. Place the banana slices in a food processor or powerful blender. Purée banana slices, scraping down the bowl as needed. Purée until the mixture is creamy and smooth. Add the peanut butter and purée to combine. Serve immediately for soft-serve ice cream consistency. If you prefer harder ice cream, place in the freezer for a few hours and then serve.

Nutritional Values Per Serving Total Calories: 153; Total Fat: 4g; Saturated Fat: 1g; Cholesterol: 0mg; Sodium: 4mg; Potassium: 422mg; Total Carbohydrates: 29g; Fiber: 4g; Sugars: 15g; Protein: 3g

Peach and Blueberry Tart

Preparation Time: 10 minutes
Cook Time: 30 minutes
Servings: 6-8

Ingredients

- 1 sheet frozen puff pastry
- 1 cup fresh blueberries
- 4 peaches, pitted and sliced
- 3 tablespoons sugar
- 2 tablespoons cornstarch
- 1 tablespoon freshly squeezed lemon juice
- Cooking spray
- 1 tablespoon nonfat or low-fat milk
- Confectioners' sugar, for dusting

Direction

1. Thaw puff pastry at room temperature for at least 30 minutes.
2. Preheat the oven to 400°F.
3. In a large bowl, toss the blueberries, peaches, sugar, cornstarch, and lemon juice.
4. Spray a round pie pan with cooking spray.
5. Unfold pastry and place on the pie pan.
6. Arrange the peach slices so they are slightly overlapping. Spread the blueberries on top of the peaches.

7. Drape pastry over the outside of the fruit and press pleats firmly together. Brush with milk.

8. Bake in the bottom third of the oven for about 30 minutes or until crust is golden.

9. Cool on a rack.

10. Sprinkle pastry with confectioners' sugar. Serve.

Nutritional Values: Per Serving Total Calories: 119; Total Fat: 3g; Saturated Fat: 1g; Cholesterol: 0mg; Sodium: 21mg; Potassium: 155mg; Total Carbohydrates: 23g; Fiber: 2g; Sugars: 15g; Protein: 1g

Berries Marinated in Balsamic Vinegar

Preparation Time: 10 minutes
Cooking Time: 0 minutes
Servings: 4

Ingredients

- 1/4 cup balsamic vinegar
- 2 tablespoons brown sugar
- 1 teaspoon vanilla extract
- 1/2 cup sliced strawberries
- 1/2 cup blueberries
- 1/2 cup raspberries
- 4 shortbread biscuits

Directions

1. Combine balsamic vinegar, vanilla, and brown sugar in a small bowl.
2. Toss strawberries with raspberries and blueberries in a bowl.
3. Pour the vinegar mixture on top and marinate for 15 minutes.
4. Serve with shortbread biscuits.

Nutritional Values: Per Serving Calories 176; Total Fat 11.9 g; Saturated Fat 1.7 g; Cholesterol 78 mg; Sodium 79 mg; Total Carbohydrates 33 g; Fiber 1.1 g; Sugar 10.3 g; Protein 13 g

Strawberries and Cream Cheese Crepes

Preparation Time: 10 minutes
Cooking Time: 10 minutes
Servings: 2

Ingredients:

- 4 tablespoons cream cheese, softened
- 2 tablespoons sifted powdered sugar
- 2 teaspoons vanilla extract
- 2 Prepared packaged crepes, each about 8 inches in diameter
- 8 strawberries, hulled and sliced

Directions

1. Preheat oven to 325°F. Grease a baking dish with cooking spray.
2. Blend cream cheese with vanilla and powder sugar in a mixer.
3. Spread the cream cheese mixture on each crepe and top with 2 tablespoons strawberries.
4. Roll the crepes and place them in the baking dish.
5. Bake for 10 minutes until golden brown.
6. Garnish as desired.
7. Serve.

Nutritional Values: Per Serving Calories 144; Total Fat 4.9 g; Saturated Fat 4.1 g; Cholesterol 11 mg; Sodium 13 mg; Total Carbohydrates 19.3 g; Fiber 1.9 g; Sugar 9.7 g; Protein 3.4 g

CONDIMENTS & SAUCES

Creamy Avocado "Alfredo" Sauce

Preparation Time: 10 minutes
Servings: 4

Ingredients

- 1 ripe avocado, peeled and pitted
- 1 tablespoon dried basil
- 1 clove garlic
- 1 tablespoon lemon juice
- 1 tablespoon olive oil
- ⅛ teaspoon salt

Directions

1. Add the avocado, basil, garlic clove, lemon juice, olive oil, and salt to a food processor. Blend until a smooth, creamy sauce forms.
2. Pour the sauce over hot pasta or vegetable noodles.

Nutritional Values: Per Serving Total Calories: 104; Total Fat: 10g; Saturated Fat: 1g; Cholesterol: 0mg; Sodium: 43mg; Potassium: 229mg; Total Carbohydrates: 4g; Fiber: 3g; Sugars: 0g; Protein: 1g

Tomato-Basil Sauce

Preparation Time: 5 minutes
Cook Time: 10 minutes
Servings: 6

Ingredients

- 2 tablespoons olive oil
- 3 garlic cloves, finely chopped
- 4 (15-ounce) cans no-salt, crushed, or chopped tomatoes
- 1 tablespoon dried basil
- Salt
- Freshly ground black pepper

Directions

1. Heat the oil in a large saucepan and sauté the garlic for about a minute until lightly browned, being careful not to burn. Add the tomatoes and basil, season with salt and pepper, and cook uncovered over medium heat for about 10 minutes.
2. Serve over pasta, grains, beans, or vegetables.

Nutritional Values: Per Serving Total Calories: 103; Total Fat: 5g; Saturated Fat: 1g; Cholesterol: 0mg; Sodium: 32mg; Potassium: 735mg; Total Carbohydrates: 15g; Fiber: 3g; Sugars: 0g; Protein: 3g

Red Pepper Pesto

Preparation Time: 20 minutes
Cook Time: 10 minutes
Servings: 3

Ingredients

- 4 red bell peppers, tops sliced off and deseeded
- 3 cups fresh basil leaves
- 3 tablespoons cashews
- 3 tablespoons grated Parmesan cheese
- 1 tablespoon olive oil
- 3 garlic cloves
- ¼ teaspoon salt

Directions

1. Place peppers in the oven on a baking sheet and turn broiler to high. Broil until peppers have blackened on all sides, turning a few times, for about 10 minutes in total.
2. Remove peppers from heat and place in a bowl. Cover with plastic wrap and set aside to cool.
3. Peel the cooled peppers. In a food processor, combine peeled peppers with the remaining ingredients. Process until mixture is smooth and resembles a pesto.

Nutritional Values: Per ¼-Cup Serving Total Calories: 50; Total Fat: 3g; Saturated Fat: 0g; Cholesterol: 1mg; Sodium: 74mg; Potassium: 185mg; Total Carbohydrates: 5g; Fiber: 1g; Sugars: 0g; Protein: 2g

Cranberry Sauce

Preparation Time: 5 minutes
Cook Time: 10 minutes,
Servings: 2

Ingredients

- ½ cup sugar
- ½ cup water
- 1 (12-ounce) package fresh or frozen cranberries
- ½ teaspoon ground cinnamon
- *Optional:* 2 tablespoons 100% orange juice

Directions

1. Combine all of the ingredients in a medium saucepan. Bring to a boil over medium-high heat, and then reduce to a simmer. Cook, stirring occasionally, until berries start to pop. Press berries against the side of the pan with a wooden spoon and continue to cook until berries are completely broken down and mixture has a jam-like consistency. Cook for about 10 minutes total.

2. Remove from heat and allow to cool. Stir in water in 1-tablespoon increments to adjust to desired consistency.

3. Serve immediately or store in the refrigerator for 10 to 14 days. You can also freeze the sauce for up to 1 to 2 months.

Nutritional Values: Per ¼ Cup Serving Total Calories: 113; Total Fat: 0g; Saturated Fat: 0g; Cholesterol: 0mg; Sodium: 0mg; Potassium: 1mg; Total Carbohydrates: 29g; Fiber: 3g; Sugars: 26g; Protein: 0g

Greek Yogurt Mayonnaise

Preparation Time: 2 minutes
Servings: 12

Ingredients

- 6 ounces nonfat or low-fat plain Greek yogurt
- 1 teaspoon apple cider vinegar
- ¼ teaspoon yellow mustard
- ¼ teaspoon hot sauce
- ¼ teaspoon freshly ground black pepper
- ¼ teaspoon paprika
- ¼ teaspoon salt

Directions

Mix all the ingredients together and blend well. Adjust seasonings to suit taste.

Nutritional Values: Per 2-Tablespoon Serving Total Calories: 8; Total Fat: 0g; Saturated Fat: 0g; Cholesterol: 0mg; Sodium: 65mg; Potassium: 2mg; Total Carbohydrates: 1g; Fiber: 0g; Sugars: 1g; Protein: 1g

Fresh Vegetable Salsa

Preparation Time: 10 minutes
Servings: 6

Ingredients

- 2 cups cored and diced bell peppers
- 2 cups diced tomatoes
- 1 cup diced zucchini
- ½ cup chopped red onion
- ¼ cup freshly squeezed lime juice
- 2 garlic cloves, minced
- 1 teaspoon freshly ground black pepper
- ¼ teaspoon salt

Directions

1. Wash the vegetables.
2. In a large bowl, combine all the ingredients. Toss gently to mix.
3. Cover and refrigerate for a few minutes to allow the flavors to blend.

Nutritional Values: Per ¼-Cup Serving Total Calories: 10; Total Fat: 0g; Saturated Fat: 0g; Cholesterol: 0mg; Sodium: 26mg; Potassium: 81mg; Total Carbohydrates: 2g; Fiber: 1g; Sugars: 1g; Protein: 0g

Tangy Barbecue Sauce

Preparation Time: 5 minutes
Servings: 2

Ingredients

- 1 (8-ounce) can no-salt tomato paste
- 2 tablespoons Dijon mustard
- 1½ tablespoons apple cider vinegar
- 1 tablespoon low-sodium soy sauce
- 2 teaspoons molasses
- 1 teaspoon garlic powder
- 1 teaspoon onion powder

Directions

1. In a medium bowl, whisk together all the ingredients until thoroughly combined.
2. Store in an airtight container in the refrigerator for up to a week.

Nutritional Values: Per ¼-Cup Serving Total Calories: 32; Total Fat: 0g; Saturated Fat: 0g; Cholesterol: 0mg; Sodium: 240mg; Potassium: 340mg; Total Carbohydrates: 7g; Fiber: 1g; Sugars: 4g; Protein: 2g

LEGUMES AND GRAINS RECIPES

Quinoa Risotto With Arugula and Parmesan

Preparation Time: 10 minutes
Cooking Time: 20 minutes
Servings: 4

Ingredients

- 1 tablespoon olive oil
- 1/2 yellow onion, chopped (about 1/2 cup)
- 1 garlic clove, minced
- 1 cup quinoa, well rinsed
- 2 1/4 cups low-sodium vegetable stock or broth
- 2 cups chopped, stemmed arugula (rocket)
- 1 small carrot, peeled and finely shredded
- 1/2 cup thinly sliced fresh shiitake mushrooms
- 1/4 cup grated Parmesan cheese
- 1/4 teaspoon salt
- 1/4 teaspoon freshly ground black pepper

Directions

1. Preheat olive oil in a saucepan on medium heat.
2. Sauté onion for 4 minutes and then stir in quinoa and garlic.
3. Cook for 1 minute before stirring in stock. Cook until it boils and then reduce the heat to a simmer.

4. Continue cooking for 12 minutes.

5. Add carrot, mushrooms, and arugula. Cook for 2 minutes.

6. Adjust seasoning with salt and pepper.

7. Garnish with cheese.

8. Serve warm.

Nutritional Values: Per Serving Calories 161; Total Fat 17.5 g; Saturated Fat 10.7 g; Cholesterol 68 mg; Sodium 763 mg; Total Carbohydrates 19.9 g; Fiber 1.3 g; Sugar 0.6 g; Protein 9.3 g

Vermicelli with Vegetables

Preparation Time: 10 minutes
Cooking Time: 15 minutes
Servings: 2

Ingredients:

- 2 teaspoons extra-virgin olive oil, divided
- 6 asparagus spears
- 4 ounces dried whole-grain vermicelli
- 1 medium tomato, chopped
- 1 tablespoon minced garlic
- 2 tablespoons chopped fresh basil
- 4 tablespoons freshly grated Parmesan, divided
- 1/8 teaspoon ground black pepper, or to taste

Directions

1. Preheat olive oil in a skillet and sauté asparagus until it's golden brown.
2. Allow them to cool and then slice into 1-inch pieces.
3. Boil vermicelli in a pot filled with water for 12 minutes. Drain and set aside.
4. Toss the pasta with 1 teaspoon olive oil, tomato, basil, garlic, asparagus, and Parmesan cheese.
5. Serve.

Nutritional Values: Calories 325; Total Fat 9.4 g; Saturated Fat 2.5 g; Cholesterol 0.4 mg; Total Carbohydrates 13.4 g; Sugar 3.1 g; Fiber 1.2 g; Sodium 310 mg; Protein 5.6 g

Yellow Lentils with Spinach and Ginger

Preparation Time: 10 minutes
Cooking Time: 15 minutes
Servings: 4

Ingredients

- 1 tablespoon olive oil
- 1 shallot, minced (about 2 tablespoons)
- 1 teaspoon ground ginger
- 1/2 teaspoon curry powder
- 1/2 teaspoon ground turmeric
- 1 cup yellow lentils, picked over, rinsed and drained
- 1 1/2 cups no-salt-added vegetable stock, chicken stock or broth
- 1/2 cup light coconut milk
- 2 cups baby spinach leaves, stemmed and chopped, or 1 cup frozen chopped spinach, thawed
- 1/2 teaspoon salt

For garnish
- 1 teaspoon white or black sesame seeds
- 1 tablespoon chopped fresh cilantro or fresh coriander

Directions

1. Preheat olive oil in a saucepan and sauté ginger and shallots with turmeric and curry powder for 1 minute.
2. Stir in lentils, coconut milk, and stock.
3. Bring to a boil. Reduce the heat to cook for 12 minutes.
4. Toast the sesame seeds in a dry pan until golden brown. Set them aside.
5. Add spinach to the lentils and cover. Cook the mixture for 3 minutes.
6. Adjust seasoning with salt.
7. Garnish with cilantro or coriander and sesame seeds.
8. Serve.

Nutritional Values: Calories 263 Total Fat 7.4 g Saturated Fat 7.1 g Cholesterol 10 mg Total Carbohydrates 15.4 g Sugar 0.7 g Fiber 2.8 g Sodium 536 mg Protein 6.2 g

Pasta with Spinach, Garbanzo Beans, and Raisins

Preparation Time: 10 minutes
Cooking Time: 10 minutes
Servings: 4

Ingredients:

- 8 ounces (about 3 cups) dry bow tie pasta
- 2 tablespoons olive oil
- 4 garlic cloves, crushed
- 1/2 of 19 ounces can of garbanzo beans, rinsed and drained
- 1/2 cup unsalted chicken broth
- 1/2 cup golden raisins
- 4 cups fresh spinach, chopped
- 2 tablespoons grated Parmesan cheese
- Cracked black peppercorns, to taste

Directions

1. Boil pasta in the pot for 12 minutes until al dente. Drain and set it aside.
2. Sauté garlic in a greased pan for 30 seconds and then add broth and garbanzo beans.
3. Cook until it is heated, then stir in spinach and raisins.
4. Let it cook for another 3 minutes.

5. Toss the pasta with the beans mixture, Parmesan cheese, and peppercorns.
6. Serve warm.

Nutritional Values: Calories 282; Total Fat 3.7 g; Saturated Fat 0.7 g; Cholesterol 0 mg; Total Carbohydrates 26.5 g; Sugar 1.4 g; Fiber 0.7 g; Sodium 141 mg; Protein 5.4 g

Do you need even more recipes?

The National Heart, Lung, and Blood Institute offers more than 180 heart-healthy recipes in its online database:

https://healthyeating.nhlbi.nih.gov/

Mayo Clinic also provides a long list of DASH-friendly recipes:

https://www.mayoclinic.org/healthy-lifestyle/recipes/dash-diet-recipes/rcs-20077146

My final request...

Being a smaller author, reviews help me tremendously!

It would mean the world to me if you could leave a review by clicking the image below which will take you directly to the review section for this book.

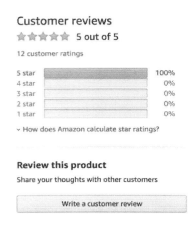

If you liked reading this book and learned a thing or two, please scan with your camera to leave your review:

It only takes 30 seconds but means so much to me! Thank you and I can't wait to see your thoughts.

Conclusion

Congratulations for getting this far of the book.

As we have seen, the Dash Diet is such a healthy weight loss and health improvement program. More people all over the world opt for this diet each day because of its multiple advantages and benefits.

Just have to follow this diet's basic principles and soon you will feel and look amazing.

Get your hands on a copy of this great Dash Diet collection and start cooking some of these delicious Dash Diet recipes.

You will love each of these recipes and you will soon become an expert in Dash Diet cooking!

So, what are you waiting for? Get started with this great lifestyle right away and have fun cooking some of these flavorful Dash Diet dishes.

At **BODY YOU DESERVE** Publishing, we strongly believe that there are a thousand ways to improve your life and health. However, there is no single recipe suitable for everyone how to do that.

We think that the best way to receive your goals is the one you can stick to and our writers will do their best to provide simple, easy to follow, step by step and realistic instructions how to do that.

At **BODY YOU DESERVE Publishing**, we strongly believe that there are a thousand ways to improve your life and health. However, there is no single recipe suitable for everyone how to do that.

We think that the best way to receive your goals is the one you can stick to and our writers will do their best to provide simple, easy to follow, step by step and realistic instructions how to do that.

To discover our best books go to link:

https://amzn.to/40B5KmZ

Or scan QR code with your camera:

Printed in Great Britain
by Amazon

26737418R00139